Medicine Made Clear

HOUSE CALLS FROM A MAINE COUNTRY DOCTOR

Michael A. LaCombe, M.D.

Illustrations by Kristina LaCombe and Gingie N. Laiho

D1707446

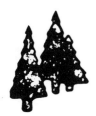

DIRIGO BOOKS
Woodstock, Maine

A Dirigo Books, Inc. Original Publication. First Edition, December 1989.

Cover Art by Gingie N. Laiho

Published in the United States by Dirigo Books, Inc., Woodstock, Maine.

Library of Congress Cataloging-in-Publication Data

LaCombe, Michael A., 1942-
    Medicine made clear: house calls from a Maine country doctor /
by Michael A. LaCombe; illustrations by Kristina LaCombe
and Gingie N. Laiho.
        p. cm.
    Bibliography: p.
    Includes index.
    ISBN 0-9623199-0-2 : $21.95
    1. Medicine, Popular. I. LaCombe, Kristina. II. Laiho, Gingie
N. III. Title.
RC81.L19   1989
613—dc20   89-16853
                                                                  CIP

Manufactured in the United States of America
10   9   8   7   6   5   4   3   2   1

For James C. Hanson

When the minds of the people are closed and wisdom is locked out, they remain tied to disease. Yet their feelings and desires should be investigated and made known, their wishes and ideas should be followed; and then it becomes apparent that those who have attained spirit and energy are flourishing and prospering, while those perish who lose their spirit and energy.

Huang Ti (2697-2597 B.C.)

Preface

This book contains advice to help you understand, treat, and prevent major medical problems. Together with that advice are stories about patients (carefully disguised) to help you understand disease. Thankfully, no one person will be asked to confront all of the disease processes discussed here. But a working knowledge of major medical problems will help you become an advocate for others as well as an advocate for yourself.

In medicine, as in other disciplines blending art and science, there are many correct ways of doing things. Rather than bore you with details by relating the pros and cons of various approaches to treatment, I have told you in this book how *I* do it. Recommendations and differences of opinion can be strikingly disparate in medicine, especially in certain gray areas such as cancer surveillance.

A word about the quality of medical care: There *is* a difference between elitism and arrogance. There is nothing wrong with demanding the highest quality available in *any* discipline. That is elitism. It is *never* arrogant to expect the best. Not in medicine, nor in law, teaching, or politics, should we ever settle for second best. This book will serve as a frame of reference for you.

This is a book for patients and for families of patients. It is not a book for doctors or other health professionals. It is meant to be a chat, a heart-to-heart talk, physician to patient—as in the old days when, on a house call, the family doctor sat at the kitchen table and told it as it was.

There are no gimmicks in this book and no quick fixes. There *is* a great deal of honest advice—but, as you already know, such honesty is not always an easy path.

The advice contained herein is based on one doctor's opinion. This advice is meant to inform you about major medical problems; it is not meant to train you to treat them. And because of space limitations, this book is not a complete compendium of all adult illness. Advice about aging, psychiatric disease, ulcer disease, and discussions of homeopathic and fringe medicine, for example, have had to be omitted.

In the appendix is a bibliography to guide you to further reading, with references by chapter. Rather than rehash what others have written about particular diets, the best recipes for bran muffins, or the mechanics of expensive running shoes, I refer you to those readings.

The book *does* welcome dialogue. It is a "house call" from a country doctor. If you have questions or ideas generated from this book, write to me at the address below. I practice in a small New England town where the mailman knows who I am and where I am— most of the time. In this day and age, that is a blessing.

Michael A. LaCombe, M.D.
Norway, Maine

Acknowledgments This book would never have been written without the help of a great many people. The author wishes to thank the following for their help:

For reviewing part or all of the manuscript for accuracy of medical information I am indebted to Drs. A. Ingrid Eriksson, Peter R. Harbage, William L. Medd, Gregory J. Riley, Donald E. Ware, Richard A. Weiner, and Michael W. Yocum.

L. Edward Willard, faculty emeritus and archivist of Hebron Academy, reviewed drafts of every chapter and assisted in editing and revision.

For library work and literature searches, the author thanks Katherine Bean. Alvin Barth did the photography used in preparation of many of the illustrations.

For her transcription, advice in editing, and indexing, I am indebted to Carol S. Plunkett.

For the fine illustrations the author thanks Kristina LaCombe and Gingie N. Laiho.

I am grateful for the guidance, criticism, and help in editing provided by Edward L. Francis, publisher, of Dirigo Books.

For her valuable advice and her patience during the writing of this book, the author thanks his wife, Dr. A. Ingrid Eriksson.

Contents

DISCLAIMER   This book is advice based on one doctor's opinions. The author urges you to discuss with your own physician the material contained in this book before you act upon it. Keep in mind that presentation of disease varies significantly. Remember also that physicians may hold widely divergent opinions on a whole variety of medical matters. The advice is intended as a reference for discussion with your doctor, not as a do-it-yourself guide. Do not hold the book in your left hand while making an appendectomy incision with your right.

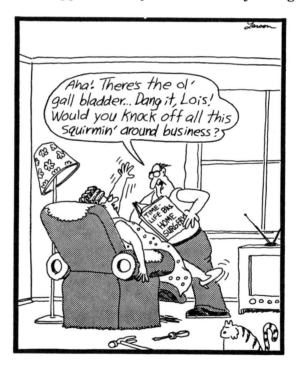

Medicine
Made
Clear

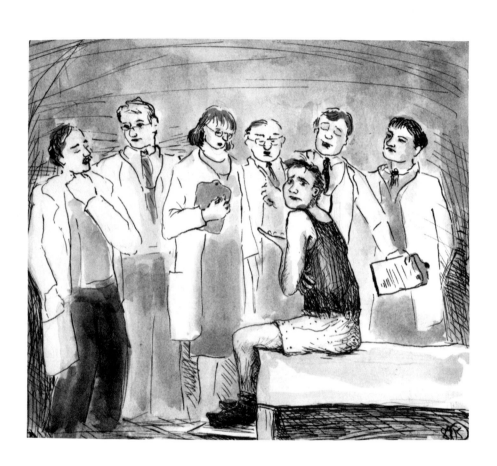

1

Who Argues for You?

"Knowledge is of two kinds. We know a subject ourselves, or we know where we can find information upon it."

Samuel Johnson
1709-1784

When do "gas pains" signal an impending heart attack? What's wrong with a penicillin shot for the flu? How many evening highballs does it take to produce cirrhosis of the liver? Which drugs are dangerous for your children under any circumstances? And can you trust *any* doctor not to prescribe these drugs?

Are all "doctors" really doctors? What's the difference between a chiropractor and an osteopath? How can you choose a doctor and tell if he or she is good? When should you switch doctors?

How often should you have a checkup? What should be "checked-up"? Why are we having so much trouble finding a cure for AIDS? Is there a moral message in the AIDS epidemic? Is there a message in *any* disease? Is oral sex abnormal? What do black bowel movements mean? Why is it so impossible to lose weight?

As a society we take great care of our lawns, our automobiles, and our television sets. Yet we know very little about our bodies. We shop for the cheapest doctor. We take blood pressure medicine for three months and then stop the drug, considering ourselves cured. We routinely ignore disturbing signs of potentially lethal—and potentially curable—disease. And we would certainly find it very difficult to answer the questions above; few doctors can answer them all. And yet, the answers should come to us as easily as do directions to the nearest Burger King.

Some societies, such as Sweden and Denmark, are quite sophisticated medically. A system of free health care works there very well. In these countries, people have learned to care for themselves. Americans do not. We eat and smoke far too much, consume far too much alcohol, and get little or no exercise. (Walk an hour each day and you will get more exercise than most Americans.)

Centuries ago, in the Great Time Before Television, people talked to one another. This was the age before the glossy magazine and the fast lane — it was a time of books and of libraries, a time when people thought for themselves and formed a point of view. There is even some evidence that in those times, doctors talked to their patients.

Why is it that we no longer talk to each other? What has happened to the long walk, the quiet chat on the veranda, the debate deep into the night at the kitchen table? And more particularly, why have we lost that moment of doctor and patient talking? Do we no longer care for each other? Have we lost our sense of family?

Today we are too willing to surrender responsibility for ourselves to others, including to our doctors. We ask others to make us thin, keep us from smoking, and give us health, too often avoiding the hard work required to do it for ourselves. Too often we allow the media to do our thinking and our feeling for us. It is not surprising that we are all in danger of losing our self-discipline.

Think for yourself. Make your own decisions. Live the life you want to live. Don't allow your life to be, as someone once said, what happens to you while you're getting ready for something else.

There is an old trick that I sometimes use with patients. I will hand a patient a sheet of paper and ask him to make two lists. On the left-hand side of the page, he is to list those activities he most cherishes: those things he loves, those pursuits which define him. When he is finished, I ask him to fold that side of the paper under and list on the right-hand side of the page all of the activities he has done today.

The two sides, of course, never match up. On the left-hand side, the side of dreams, he has listed all of those moments that are the "sweeter banquets of the mind," moments such as reading a book, or talking with a friend, or listening to music, or walking in the woods with someone. And on the right-hand side, he has listed those trivialities on which we too often squander our lives.

WHAT THIS BOOK IS

And so we come to this book. This is a book about taking care of yourself, about taking responsibility for yourself, and about caring for one another. It is an opportunity to talk to a doctor, because that's what patients want after all. This is a book about communication, and about shared responsibility. It is a book of information about ourselves, on how to take care of ourselves, on how to help doctors take care of us, and on how to care for doctors. It is a book on how to stop and smell the flowers and on how to increase our chances of being there when the flowers arrive next spring.

What follows is one doctor's view of what makes up good doctors and good patients. It is a discussion of what is experienced with illness and how you can recognize the more common diseases and ailments afflicting us. It is a book about how to become your own best advocate for your health and how to make the right decisions in that regard. The anecdotes contained herein are fictionalized encounters from twenty years of practice in America and Europe, as well as in that very special country, Maine. It is a book of reference, when, for example, there is a question about breast cancer or heart disease. It is a book to lead you further in your reading about your concerns, by way of the Bibliography contained in the Appendix.

WHAT THIS BOOK IS NOT

This book is not a substitute for a visit to your doctor. It is neither a health manual nor an exhaustive compendium of diseases and their treatments. It is a point of reference for discussion to be used to help you think for yourself, to talk to one another, and to your doctor and to help you make intelligent decisions about your health. As a reference for discussion, this book may be very helpful as a companion at your visit to the doctor. You may, for example, say to your doctor, "I want to start an exercise program, and this book says that I should have a treadmill exercise test first. What do you think?"

DO YOU WANT A DOCTOR OR AN INSTITUTION?

I have a friend with a terrible disease. When he was first diagnosed as having leukemia, because he was a physician, he had the physician's facility with medical literature, the physician's accessibility to the best university minds, and the physician's inside knowledge of what was best to do and how and when to do it.

For his disease, bone marrow transplantation offered the only hope for cure. My friend researched the results of America's various bone marrow transplantation centers. He found the best leukemia specialist on the East Coast and consulted with her about what to do and where to go for treatment. He consulted as well with his brother, who was a cancer specialist. For his bone marrow transplantation, he chose a large university center in the Northeast.

In this vast hospital specializing only in cancer treatment, my friend had a doctor to admit him to the hospital, a second doctor to examine his bone marrow, a third doctor to direct his chemotherapy, a fourth doctor to administer his chemotherapy, another doctor to remove his spleen, and still another doctor to analyze his spleen. There was a doctor to direct the whole separate procedure of bone marrow transplantation, another doctor to perform the transplantation, and doctors to monitor its progress. He had a doctor to administer the total body radiation therapy he required and another doctor to treat infections that might result. He had a doctor ready to minister to his psyche, should he need it, and doctors standing by to meet any complications that might arise.

Yet, my physician-friend had *no* doctor. He was a patient of the institution. He had a great deal of difficulty finding out who was in charge, who directed his care.

Who argues for you? Who will bang on the doors of the inner sanctums for you, give you the accessibility and knowledge you need, ask the right questions for you, get the right answers you need, and help you feel in control? In this new age of managed medical care, the public is being sold a bill of goods in order to contain health care costs. You are being offered *institutions* to care for you at the expense of having your own personal physician. Unless you can become your own advocate, you may find yourself someday, as did my friend, wondering who is in charge.

To argue intelligently for yourself, you will need some of my friend's medical sophistication. This book will begin to provide that for you. You will need a well-chosen personal physician to act as your advocate in your stead. This book will tell you how to find him or her. Armed with some medical knowledge and some wisdom about choices available and assisted by your personal physician whom you trust, you can begin to pick your way through the bewildering maze of American medicine. Remember, there are many correct ways of doing things. Excellent physicians have different philosophies and different approaches to the same illness. All approaches may be correct. Medicine is not an exact science and, as long as we have human beings for patients and doctors, it never will be. But you do need some medical sophistication and a doctor whom you trust. That is what this book is for.

I will tell you what you cannot do: When you are already deep in crisis and full of emergency, you cannot, on a moment's notice, bang on the doors of the best and the brightest and expect to be seen. Even if you are fortunate enough to have money and power, you may find that in using that power to open doors for you, you will have inconvenienced a very busy physician. You may thus begin your relationship with him or her laced with a heavy tone of resentment.

I will tell you what else you cannot do: You cannot expect your nonphysician friends, when you are deep in crisis, to help you very much at all in sorting out medical options, choices of therapy, or selections of physicians. Medicine is a queer business. It rapidly becomes confused with magic, gimmickery, and quackery and is heavily shrouded in myth. Your friends may be biased and ill-informed about choices in medical therapy.

I will tell you what else you cannot do: You cannot make a silk purse out of a sow's ear. If you make an uninformed choice of physicians and find yourself bound to a physician who is uninformed himself, no amount of screaming and pleading will make him into an Albert Schweitzer.

Also, there is a danger in taking *too* much control. Physicians continually meet patients who "doctor shop." They do this because of denial or mistrust or because of a fear of relinquishing control at all. I had a patient recently with significant heart disease. He was a fit elderly man who complained of chest pain with exertion. He could neither split nor stack his wood, nor mow his lawn, nor prune his apple trees. Routine tests in our small country hospital revealed that he had severe coronary artery disease, a significant blockage of his heart's circulation.

I recommended medication immediately and scheduled him for urgent study of his coronary arteries at a nearby large medical center. He said that he would think about it. He read extensively about heart disease.

They had better doctors in Boston, he decided. He consulted them by phone. He decided he would like to have his X-rays done in Boston. And besides, the Veterans Hospital there would be cheaper since he was a veteran. That was reasonable, I responded. I would see that it was scheduled. I called the physicians at a Veterans Hospital in Boston and presented his case over the phone. I sent his records and made an appointment for him to be admitted to that hospital.

He backed out. He would think about it some more. He read more articles on heart disease. His wife had talked to her doctor in a neighboring, larger town. They both consulted with him. There were, it seemed, conflicting opinions. He would think about it some more.

It has now been a year since he has begun cogitating about what to do with himself. In the meantime because of the nature of his heart disease, he has run the very real risk of sudden death.

Your body is not some magical machine that is hermetically sealed and never wanting maintenance. It is both more wonderful than a machine and more fragile. It demands of you a knowledge of how it works, an understanding of what might go wrong, and informed anticipation of problems early in disease. It asks that you undergo certain periodic inspections, preventative maintenance, and it begs you not to take risks. It asks that you find a bright knowledgeable mechanic to minister to it, someone as assiduously selected as the repairman for your stereo equipment.

Expect and demand quality. You are never arrogant in doing so. There are some doctors in practice who are poorly trained, or who use out-dated medical knowledge, or who are even consumed by greed. But they are few — contrary to what the media would have you believe. Most physicians are hard-working, dedicated human beings who still, in these times, find it rather easy to care for their fellow human beings.

Find the doctor right for you. That is what our next chapter will help you do.

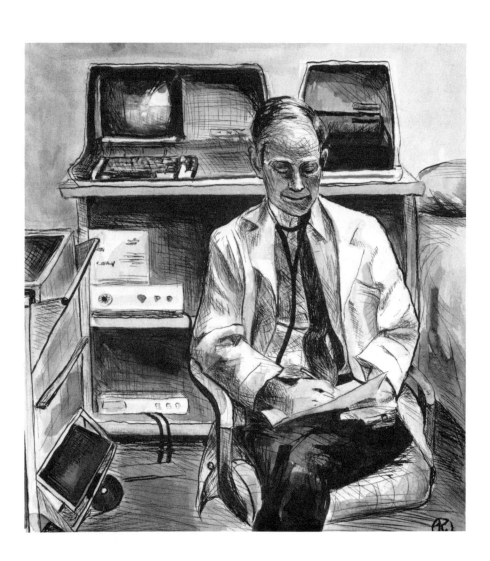

2

Finding the Perfect Doctor

"Forty years of teaching have taught me this: that it is relatively easy to become a competent specialist, but it is much more difficult to become a good doctor — and it takes much longer."

William Doolin

Suppose for a moment you've been charged with murder. Your neighbor's body, together with the bodies of his three pitbull terriers, has been found in the jumble of junked cars on his front lawn. His electric guitar and power amps are smashed with a vengeance. Somehow the authorities believe you might have a motive.

You were photographing wildflowers near the town dump. Alone. That's your alibi. Maybe you'd better get a lawyer. You'll get the best of course, and you won't start by looking in the Yellow Pages. You might even call a few lawyer acquaintances to get a recommendation. Your life is on the line.

When, after a thorough, meticulous search, you have found the perfect lawyer, you will trust him implicitly. You won't lie to him, you'll stick to the pertinent facts and use his time wisely. You'll do exactly as he tells you, and lest he lose interest, you'll be careful not to bore him, nor bother him with minutiae. It is *your* neck. The police are talking about "the chair," and you have a very clear idea of what is at stake. The specter of a death sentence does give one a sense of purpose.

Why do we never approach a doctor's visit this way, but rather act as though we were dropping off the old Chevy at the local garage?

THE BUSINESS OF DENIAL

Why *is* there this difference? Why do we usually minister to our pets more properly than to ourselves, carefully measuring their nutritionally balanced diet while our own suppers of pork and fries simmer in the deep fryer?

It has to do with denial. We do not glimpse the "grim reaper" often enough, hardly ever see him clearly, and often never at all, even when we are dying. We wish to believe we will live forever — forever young and fit and disease-free. We want our doctors to tell us only that we are immortal, confirming what we want to hear. The obligatory checkup becomes one item on a long list, just above picking up the laundry.

This denial can be fierce and can cause us to behave in strange ways. It is said that it takes at most six months for the mind to forget (or deny) the most severe of lessons. In that time, a man who has suffered a devastating heart attack with its collapse and pain, cardiac arrest and resuscitation, furrowed brows and weeping families — within that time, he will be smoking again.

Or this denial will work another way, causing the patient to believe that disease is extraneous, foreign to the human condition, introduced by an attitude of mind, or even by the doctor. In its mildest form, this denial surfaces in the belief that if "I don't go to the doctor, she won't find anything." We have all felt this way. If I don't look, it isn't there. The whining fanbelt, the halting engine, the fleeting chest pain — ignore them all and they will go away. Denial of disease can take on bizarre proportions.

Let me tell you about one patient. . . . This man semi-retired to Maine at just about the time I started practice here. He would become for me the most personal Jonah I would ever know. Our relationship began with his heart attack. His hospitalization was complicated: a heart catheter, dangerous heart rhythms, a temporary pacemaker. He survived. On his day of discharge he said he hoped he'd never see me again. I could accept that. He wasn't leaving a three-star restaurant.

A year later his wife made him come in for a checkup. (This is the usual reason men get checkups.) During the examination I found that he had diabetes.

"I never had a sick day in my life until I met you," he said disgustedly.

Two years later I found in him a very early, asymptomatic rectal cancer. He wound up with a colostomy and a cure. He focused on the colostomy, blaming the cancer on me.

"You're the one who found it!" he said. He believed, of course, that I had put it there.

A few years later he developed a fatal heart-valve infection that took his life before a cancer of the esophagus could kill him. Before he died, he said:

I never should have come to Maine. I have been sick ever since I met you.

He abhorred seeing me. It was his wife who always made him come. I was never his favorite person. Yet, without good medicine, he never would have met his grandson. He had believed he'd live forever. It was his wife who was not convinced. And though it always seemed to hang over him, he never saw that Great Inevitability we all are inclined to deny.

Contending With Denial

How can you improve your chances of meeting your grandchildren? Visit the sick. Bury your friends. Don't deny the passing of your loved ones. Don't deny your own mortality. Use this book and the information in it to understand your own body and how that machine can malfunction. Use this book to expand communication between yourself and your doctor. And most essential, as though your life depended upon it, search for the best doctor you can find.

FINDING A DOCTOR

You will start by looking for an **internist.** (An internist specializes in the diagnosis and nonsurgical treatment of adult diseases. An intern, on the contrary, is the now-outdated term for a doctor in his first year of hospital training after medical school.) If it's your children who need a doctor, you will be looking for a **pediatrician.** In some instances, for both adult and child medical care, you will be searching for a **family practitioner.** More about why later. Start looking by asking around. Begin with the realtor. Ask at your first few get-togethers. Call the Visiting Nurses' Association. Call the director of nursing at the local hospital. Remember you are looking for an *internist,* not for someone's favorite doctor. Ask for a favorite doctor and you'll get a lot of subjective evaluations — and the names of specialists you don't need . . . yet. And remember, keep your own mortality in mind. Your life is in the balance. Remember, they've found your neighbor strangled with loudspeaker cable, and the jury knows you hate heavy metal rock.

Soon the same names will begin to surface. You now have a list. Now limit your choices by looking for an internist who is *board-certified* — that is, has passed a certifying examination in internal medicine. The hospital's administrator can give you this information, or you can call or write the American College of Physicians (see Bibliography), the national organization of internists. *Board-eligible* is not the same as *board-certified*. *Board-eligible* implies waiting to take the board examination, but that is true only for young internists fresh from a training program. *Board-eligible* also may mean something quite different: an inability to pass the certifying examinations, for example.

Rx————————————————————————

Finding a Good Internist

- Start your list by asking around town for internists.
- Ask the Visiting Nurses' Association.
- Ask the director of nursing at the local hospital.
- Pare down your list by limiting it to board-certified internists.
- Find out about board-certification through the hospital administrator or the American College of Physicians.
- Remember, board-eligible does not necessarily mean board-certified.
- Remember, you are looking for an internist, not someone's favorite doctor.

Making the Appointment

You now have a list of board-certified internists. When do you call for the first appointment? When you are sick? Will a hidden cancer make you feel sick? Well then, when your husband or wife makes you go? No. You call now. The best doctors are extremely busy. You'll get an appointment in a few months if you call for one today. Or you will find that her practice will be closed, that she is accepting no new patients, and you will be left asking her receptionist for a recommendation. Then you'll need to consult your list and start the search over. But this search is important. You are beginning a relationship now for that time down the road when your own mortality becomes painfully obvious.

You should be given a lengthy first appointment. The internist will want to get to know you, *all* of you —all of your medical history, your family history, your quirks and idiosyncrasies — and he or she will want to perform a thorough physical examination (more on that in Chapter Four). This will take more than fifteen minutes. It may take more than one visit. The first appointment will cost you about the equivalent of ten cartons of cigarettes or ten fifths of good Scotch.

A story . . . . Every doctor can remember the first few appointments he or she has in private practice. In those days, I was banging around the office, flipping through magazines, and wondering if I would ever meet the mortgage payments, when another doctor in town called and asked if I could help him with a patient.

"Of course, send him right over!" I yelled.

The patient arrived. So eager was I to be working, actually working, that I ushered him into the examining room myself, sat down, and went into great detail about the philosophy of the practice, how to get a hold of me in an emergency, what kind of health maintenance programs I advocated in my office — this sort of thing. Finally easing up, I asked him what was the matter. He looked at me oddly and said:

> *It's not me. It's my Great Dane. He has asthma. Doc Mathers said maybe you could give us the right dose of medication.*

Internist or Super-Specialist?

Why not save time and cash, skip the internist, and instead go directly to the super-specialist? For one reason, *you* are not a diagnostician. Neither you nor your best friend know what kind of super-specialist you might need. You cannot be expected to know whether that new lump on your body should be seen by a surgeon or by a cancer specialist. You need someone you *trust,* who is trained to know, to direct you.

This brings up the business of *wants* versus *needs.* We *want* a kindly old physician, partridge-plump, with wire-rimmed glasses, blue eyes, a roll-top desk, and journals scattered about everywhere. His phone never rings, he's never interrupted, and he sits and talks to us for hours. He takes a blood pressure reading, looks at our hands, slips his stethoscope down inside the shirt, and tells us everything is just fine. He charges ten dollars for the visit, and we step weightless out into the sunlight.

What we *need* is a doctor who is hunting for disease and, more importantly, committed to preventing disease. But we get this want-need business quite mixed up. We *want* a doctor like the one on television and unfortunately may end up getting one. We are relieved when our doctor smokes or is fat, because that gives us license to practice the same vices. It's human nature. We want everything to be easy, free of stress, and comforting. But a doctor's office can't always be that way. The doctor-patient relationship is like any other relationship: It gets better as it matures over time. The *comfort* value of having a *competent* personal physician is inestimable — many times patients' lives are "uncomplicated" by reassurance and support from a personal physician. Yet that reassurance always must be based upon competence.

The first reason you don't run directly to a specialist is that you can't tell what you need. The second reason is that the specialist may not be able to tell you what you need either. The subspecialist in internal medicine (see Table 2-1) is highly trained in his or her discipline and *usually is only partially trained in general adult medicine*. Because of a concentration in one specific area of internal medicine, his or her knowledge of the rest of internal medicine becomes rusty with disuse.

A story . . . . In residency days, we doctors-in-training would preen ourselves for attending rounds. It was the high point of our day when the respected teacher would come to the medical ward, make rounds with us on our patients, dispense pearls of wisdom, and, with the more complicated patients, give us sound advice on management. We had at that time a bright young cardiologist (now nationally preeminent in her specialty) as our attending physician. We had prepared

TABLE 2-1   Subspecialists in Internal Medicine and What They Treat

- **Allergist-immunologist:** Allergies; diseases of the immune system (e.g., lupus, scleroderma)
- **Cardiologist:** Heart disease, high blood pressure
- **Dermatologist:** Skin disease
- **Endocrinologist:** Diseases of the endocrine glands (e.g., diabetes, thyroid disease, reproductive diseases)
- **Gastroenterologist:** Diseases of the intestines, liver, and bile system
- **Hematologist:** Blood diseases (e.g., anemias, leukemias)
- **Infectious disease specialist:** Diseases caused by bacteria, viruses, fungi, protozoa
- **Nephrologist:** Kidney disease, high blood pressure
- **Neurologist:** Diseases of the nervous system
- **Oncologist:** Cancers of all types
- **Pulmonologist:** Lung disease, diseases of the respiratory system
- **Rheumatologist:** Arthritis, diseases of the bones and joints

a "great case" for her: an elderly man with a terribly diseased heart valve with its attendant murmurs and intriguing sounds. She would be excited, we knew. The patient also had an odd lung disorder, blood in his bowel movements, and prostate cancer. His blood count was extremely low, his chest X-ray looked horrendous, and his spleen was enlarged. Our respected specialist listened to us as we presented the patient's history and physical findings, then stepped back and said:

What this guy needs is a doctor.

There is an additional reason not to seek out a super-specialist for initial care, and it is this: When all you have is a hammer, everything looks like a nail.

When you complain of chest pain to a cardiologist, he thinks of angina; the pulmonologist thinks embolism; the surgeon, a dissecting aneurysm; the oncologist, cancer; and the psychiatrist, a symptom of hysteria.

What About Other Generalists?

Now let's talk about the thornier question. This is an issue hotly debated, and has to do with the whole philosophy of medicine, disease, and treatment. Most physicians who become board-certified in a given discipline spend three to five years after medical school in training. They may spend those years seeing and doing a little bit of everything or, at the other extreme, they may concentrate on one discipline only — for example, psychiatry.

A general internist spends his or her three or four years of residency in the diagnosis and nonsurgical treatment of diseases of adults. The pediatrician does likewise for children. During those years the doctor in training spends varying amounts of time in the medical subspecialties listed in Table 2-1, and most of this experience is involved in caring for sick in-hospital patients in those subspecialties. This well-trained internist may never learn to lance a boil or remove a wen, but can confidently examine a patient and is trained to know when things go wrong.

The board-certified family practitioner, on the other hand, usually spends three years of training after medical school rotating through the various medical disciplines, working for six months each in obstetrics, general surgery, pediatrics, emergency medicine, psychiatry, as well as in internal medicine. (The accent in the training program for family practitioners is on taking care of healthy people on an out-patient basis.) The well-trained family practitioner *can* drain a boil, deliver a baby, and hear a heart murmur. And a well-trained family practitioner knows when to refer — early, and often. Family practitioners, those physicians board-certified in family medicine, specialize in preventative medicine, early recognition of disease, and family dynamics. Because of their training, family practitioners are usually better at dealing with families and their reactions to significant illness. Board-certified internists on the other hand have considerably more training in intensive, interventional diagnostic, and therapeutic medicine.

General Internist Versus Family Practitioner

When should you choose one over the other? You should recognize first of all that in many areas of the country, especially in rural areas, you may not have a choice. These days, the specialty of internal medicine is training fewer general internists who do primary medical care. The subspecialties of internal medicine, with their high salaries and glamorous university settings, attract many internists in training, depleting the ranks of primary care general internists. Today, America needs about 2,500 more internists and yet has too many cardiologists by about 5,500. Especially in rural areas, primary care internal medicine may be primarily practiced by family medicine practitioners. Choose a *board-certified* family practitioner and you will not go wrong. And remember, this rule should always pertain: *When significant illness strikes, and especially if that illness is complicated and requires hospitalization, then the internist, internist/subspecialist, or surgeon should take over.*

Family Practitioner Versus General Practitioner

People *want* a family doctor. People want one doctor for the whole family — one doctor to deliver the babies, to remove a mole, and to treat Mom's pneumonia. But why do people want a family doctor? Television is expert in creating wants. The image of the doctor on television is commonly the image of the family doctor. And there is a certain nostalgia for the old-time general practitioner.

Let's examine the old-time general practitioner: He could remove a diseased gallbladder. He treated pneumonias with one of a few antibiotics at his disposal. When the family was stressed, he was there to counsel and to hold the hand. He applied the cast, removed a cataract, and even gave his own anesthesia while doing so.

Once upon a time, the general practitioner had his heyday. He was a phenomenon. I was lucky enough to meet one such incredible person. This man, with a smattering of training in all of the disciplines, took his gifts to the wilds of Alaska. He worked in a small, fourteen-bed hospital in the tundra as the community's only physician. He did everything, from pinning hips to treating congestive heart failure to managing meningitis in a child. When I asked him about his practice — what was most challenging — he said that he loved it all, but I remember his rolling his eyes and saying:

But I'll tell you, Doc, when you're taking out cataracts without an assistant, and giving your own anesthesia at the same time, you are one hell of a busy man!

His day, and the day of that brand of general practitioner, is past.

A general practitioner may have only one year of postgraduate training after medical school, with three months each in medicine, pediatrics, surgery, and obstetrics-gynecology before hanging out the shingle. There is no law requiring a general practitioner to have any more training than that. And organized medicine has always been poor in regulating what doctors may or may not do in practice. There's *no* regulation specifying a minimum amount of training necessary, for example, to manage a patient in diabetic crisis. Frightening, isn't it? That is part of the reason why we are burdened with this malpractice crisis. The lawyers can be blamed only in part. Medicine has done a notoriously poor job of policing its profession, and now it suffers the consequences. Or, as Robert Frost was fond of saying: "Provide, provide . . . or someone will provide for you."
A general practitioner is *not* a family practitioner. The general practitioner has no board-certification and has far less training than the family practitioner. These two primary care practitioners should never be confused. They often *are* confused. General practitioners may advertise, in the yellow pages or elsewhere, that they "specialize" in family medicine. This does not

TABLE 2–2   Generalists (Primary Care Physicians)

- **Chiropractor:** A practitioner who is a graduate of a school of the chiropractic, which teaches a system of mechanical therapeutics that attributes diseases to disorders of the spine and treats them with manipulation of the vertebrae in order to relieve pressure on the nerves in the spinal column.

- **Family Practitioner:** A physician who has completed a three year approved residency in family practice and who may practice any or all of the following: internal medicine, pediatrics, obstetrics, office gynecology, minor outpatient and office surgery.

- **General Practitioner:** A physician who has one or more years of hospital training (residency) beyond medical school and whose practice is similar to that of a family practitioner.

- **Internist:** A physician who has four to five years of training after four years of medical school specializing in the diagnosis and nonsurgical treatment of diseases of adults.

- **Osteopath:** A physician who is a graduate of an approved school of osteopathic medicine (as opposed to medical school), which is based on the theory that the normal body when in correct adjustment is capable of making its own remedies against toxic conditions. The osteopathic physician relies on physical, hygienic, medicinal, and surgical measures, as well as osteopathic manipulation (osteopathic physicians may be internists, pediatricians, family practitioners, general practitioners, cardiologists, etc.).

- **Pediatrician:** A physician who has three to four years of training after four years of medical school specializing in the medical and hygienic care of children and the diseases of children.

make them family medicine practitioners with board certification. If all else fails, you can call the nearest medical school and ask for the Department of Family Medicine. Usually they can give you the names of physicians in your area who are board-certified in family medicine.

If you are young and healthy, between the ages of eighteen and forty, and have no significant medical problems and you prefer the family medicine practitioner with his expertise in family dynamics and preventative medicine, you will do well to find a well-trained board-certified family pracitioner. Well-trained family practitioners are excellent out-patient physicians for healthy young adults. Remember our proviso, however: If you become seriously ill and hospitalized you will require consultation with an internist, internist/subspecialist, or surgeon. A competent board-certified family practitioner will not have a quarrel with that. If you are young and suffer from chronic disease, diabetes or heart disease for example, it may be more advisable for you to start with an internist, because you may unfortunately be hospitalized with some regularity.

Suppose you are a young, healthy woman and you have found a wonderful gynecologist whom you wish to have care for you. Fine. You will get a well-performed breast and pelvic examination and a properly performed Pap smear. But you should still see an internist or family practitioner every five years for the remainder of the physical examination until you are forty and then perhaps more often than that.

Once you have found your doctor, how do you tell whether he or she is right for you? Is there such a thing as "the care and feeding of a doctor?" How can you be a "good patient" so that your encounters with your doctor are most meaningful? How do you give a good history? How can a "bad patient" jeopardize his or her care? These are some of the subjects of the next chapter.

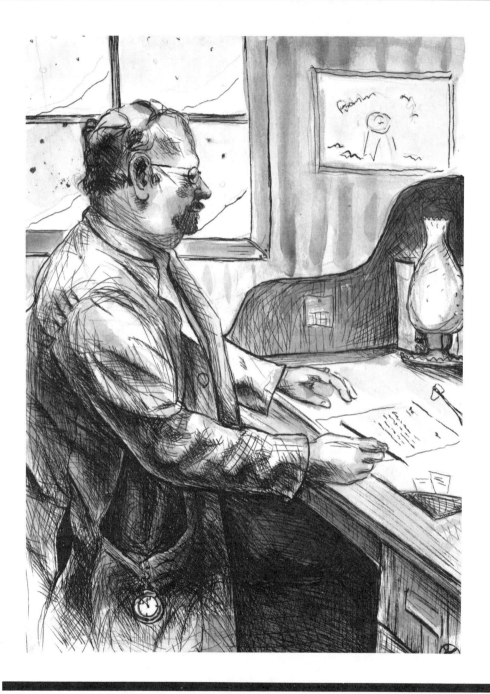

3

Patients and Doctors: What's Best

"What I call a good patient is one who, having found a good physician, sticks to him till he dies ... once in a while you'll have a patient of sense, born with the gift of observation, from whom you may learn something."

Oliver Wendell Holmes
(1809-1894)

Ages ago on that first bright, clear day in medical school, someone handed us an essay on how to be a good doctor. That was at a time before we even worried about that sort of thing. It just wasn't a concern. We were simply going to *be* good doctors. But there it was, the essay. The last sentence was unforgettable:

> *One of the essential qualities of the clinician is interest in humanity, for the secret of the care of the patient is in caring for the patient.*

Love your patients and (if you have good training as well) being a good doctor will take care of itself. And that is the best yardstick I have found to measure a good doctor: whether your doctor really cares for you, in a loving sort of way. That is, after all, the essence of the bond between doctor and patient. A mutual feeling of love, of warmth, of friendship cements a doctor-patient relationship like few others. If your doctor has good training as well, you are both set for life.

The previous chapter gave you an approach to finding a well-trained doctor. But a well-trained doctor may not necessarily be a good doctor, and the assessment of whether a doctor is good or not is a whole lot more personal than the size of his fee, the glowing reports of his patients, the number of cars parked in the front of his office, or the number of diplomas hanging on the wall. I really believe, you see, that if a person is well-trained in whatever he does and if he also cares, he will do a good job.

None of us is perfect when it comes to judging people. And it can be especially difficult, when you're seriously ill, to decide whether your doctor does really care. And so to some practical matters. Let's consider some practice styles and character types. The occupational diseases of doctors are many, but there are two problems that may especially affect patients: *Arrogance* and *extreme skepticism* arise out of the power the physician gets from his social standing, income, respect in the community, and awesome responsibility. But power corrupts, as we all know, possibly driving any doctor to extremes of pride and detachment.

PRACTICE STYLES

The doctor-patient relationship spans the spectrum from authoritarianism to anarchy. Both the patient and the doctor are responsible for where their relationship falls along that spectrum. A rigidly **authoritarian relationship** will result from a doctor's arrogance and from the excessive dependence of a patient. Rarely is this type of relationship beneficial to the patient, although certain psychotherapies do demand this approach to accomplish anything at all. At the other extreme, a doctor's excessive self-doubt and skepticism can result in an **anarchic relationship,** which also will seldom benefit the sick patient. Best is somewhat to the left of center, a liberal, **mutual partnership** with some authority retained by the doctor. This style gives some responsibility to the patient for his or her own care, relying upon the properly educated patient to report symptoms and changes in body habits — relying on the patient to point out, for example, a subtle but definite breast lump appearing during a patient's own monthly breast examination.

For many reasons patients are uncomfortable with this type of relationship and seek the authoritarian relationship of the extreme right. We've hinted at the why of this — that is, how we avoid taking responsibility for ourselves, how we search for a magic pill to make the fat dissolve and the cigarettes disappear. Patients also mistakenly believe that a rigid, decisive, arrogant doctor who makes decisions for them is the best kind of doctor to have. But the patient's extreme dependence on such a figure obviates any responsibility for self. How can this be beneficial?

When we were in training, an attending physician at our university hospital was notorious for his authoritarian approach. If we wrote in the patient's orders "15 cc of such-and-such," he would correct it, crossing out our orders, and writing in "10 cc" or "20 cc" or make some miniscule change to maintain, we surmised, his control. His patients were not to make a move without his knowledge or without his consent. Could they take an aspirin for a headache? Could they go for a ride in the country? Is a temperature of 99 degrees Fahrenheit a fever? There was a nosebleed yesterday, lasting five

minutes or so. Did he want to know? My recollection of
him, or rather my mental picture of his office door, is
vivid still. His door was always plastered with telephone
messages taped to it — completely covered, like scales
on a fish — so that when he returned from rounds on the
wards, he had this to greet him everyday. This was his
reward for his authoritarian style.

There are some patients who search for an anarchic
type of relationship. These are the doctor shoppers, the
dabblers in various kinds of fringe medicine. They too
are searching for magic. A doctor who participates in
this kind of arrangement ignores one of the true
mysteries of medicine, a mystery acknowledged since
before Hippocrates, that some authority is necessary
for healing.

That kind of authority can be of great comfort for
the dying. As I write this, I have been running between
my office and the hospital to hold the hand of a dying
man who looks at me and wants to know if everything
will be all right. I nod and tell him that everything is
fine, and hearing this, he can close his eyes and sleep for
a while.

Remember though, that in the main, when you
judge practice styles, you want to be taught, not told.

DOCTOR TYPES TO AVOID

The two occupational diseases of doctors — arrogance
and skepticism — produce certain character types and
certain practice styles. Since you've made your search
following the advice in Chapter Two, you have a list of
well-trained, well-credentialed physicians. You should
now pick from that list a physician who can keep both
his pride and self-doubt in harness (whenever he finds
the time). A caveat: As both patient and doctor myself, I
have encountered hundreds of physicians but only a
small handful of the following character-types. However, you need to know about them.

The **Shirking Procastinator,** endowed with an
excessive amount of skepticism and self-doubt, prefers
the anarchic type of doctor-patient relationship. He will
prescribe the medication you wish. You need only ask.

He will tend to avoid examining you unless you have a specific complaint, and you will note that he prefers rose-colored glasses. This group has a subspecies, the *Guileful Guilt-provoker*. Burdened with self-doubt, he avoids any responsibility for the patient and, when pressed, tends to treat the patient by the provocation of guilt, viewing the patient's complaints as the patient's own fault. This type in the extreme — and I am furious when I encounter him — is the physician who tells the cancer patient that she is responsible for her own disease (more about that later)! Another subspecies in this group is the *Artful Dodger*. She skillfully avoids encounters with patients and families and avoids the necessary explanations of illness that a patient requires. But don't confuse the Artful Dodger with the busy doctor who must necessarily employ the help of nurses, nurse practitioners, and physicians' assistants to deal with the more routine tasks of filling prescriptions, diagnosis and treatment, and patient education. Still, when you have what you believe is an emergency, you should always be able to talk to your doctor. Furthermore, questions that are highly confidential should be discussed only with your doctor, as is your right.

The **Arrogant Overweener** is at the authoritarian end of the spectrum. With an abundance of pride, this doctor displays offensive superiority and excessive self-importance, is angered by second opinions (even wounded by them), and will not brook any question of his judgment, much less question that judgment himself. The *Petulent Prima Donna*, loving praise, hating criticism, and ever temperamental, is in this group. He can never be made to wait, but will allow others to wait for him. The Arrogant Overweener finds it impossible to permit the patient to take responsibility for himself. His bristling response to the question "Doctor, what would you think of a second opinion?" identifies him.

Here comes the **Eristic Jouster,** bent on self-promotion, adored by attorneys. His standard approach is to disparage other doctors, other therapeutic maneuvers. "You got to me just in time," he says. "*He* did *that* to you?" he asks. "I can't *believe* he prescribed that medicine," he pronounces. These are his familiar songs. This self-serving stance stimulates litigation but, to his dismay, the Eristic Jouster, because he may have the deepest pocket of all, often finds himself deeply embroiled in those lawsuits he himself has stimulated.

A story . . . . a few years ago, I had a throat condition that caused me to lose my voice and worry about malignancy. I sought the advice of a specialist, a good physician in a nearby city. Unable to make a diagnosis, he referred me on, admitting that he was perplexed with the condition (such an admission is indicative of a doctor not ruled by pride). My wife and I made the long trip to the Boston specialist. The specialist, an Arrogant Overweener as I would discover, permitted his residents to examine me but never did examine me himself, spending most of the fifteen minutes of our appointment on his telephone in the examining room. He would not allow my wife, a physician, to be in the room with me. And he did not have time for our questions. I was abusing my voice, he said, talking too much to my patients. (I guessed that he would never have my problem.) My condition worsened. I was reduced to a whisper and began to think of other jobs. In desperation I found another Boston specialist. He examined me carefully, had his resident do the same, and then examined me again. He then smiled and said:

I know exactly what you have.

I asked him why the other doctors hadn't diagnosed my condition. (This is the moment the Eristic Jouster lives for!) My doctor smiled and said:

You have a rare condition, and besides, I wasn't there.

I wasn't there, he said. He wouldn't joust. He had no need to promote himself. He had made a diagnosis and was concerned about me. That was his purpose. No other agenda. Such an attitude in a physician is so becoming, but jousters never seem to realize it.

Certain patient-types prefer certain of these character-types. Hypochondriacs love the Shirking Procastinator, who will give the hypochondriac whatever he asks for: whatever test, whatever medicine, whatever surgical procedure. Angry, litigious patients seem attracted to the Eristic Jouster and dependent, passive patients obviously prefer the Arrogant Overweener.

It is well to note that all of us as doctors have a little of each of these character-types within us, and have to contend with them everyday. I have myself avoided patients and their families, frequently tripped over my pride, and have, I am sorry to say, been guilty myself of jousting. Most doctors would admit the same.

PATIENT ROLES TO AVOID

Patients cannot be faulted for their reaction to illness; it is a part of the disease. But we can all, nevertheless, behave quite badly as patients. At the time when I was convinced I had cancer, I wallowed in self-pity and found myself frequently wishing I could give my disease to someone else. Good doctors realize the humanness in this bad behavior and can excuse it. Still, just as there are bad character types among doctors, there are also those dreadful patients we like to avoid.*

The **Dependent Clinger** may or may not be ill, but does have an insatiable need and views the physician as inexhaustible. Dependent Clingers "...escalate from mild and appropriate requests for reassurance to repeated, incarcerating cries for explanation, affection, analgesics, sedatives, and all forms of attention imaginable," according to Groves. They display an excessive amount of gratitude in contrast to the second type, the **Entitled Demander.** Entitled Demanders show aggression rather than gratitude in an attempt to control and exhaust the physician: "Either you meet me in the emergency room in thirty minutes, or I'm calling my

*Comments and terms in this section are taken, by permission, from James E. Groves, "Taking Care of the Hateful Patient," *New England Journal of Medicine,* Vol. 298, April 20, 1978, p. 883.

lawyer." The Entitled Demander has a "sense of innate and magical entitlement to everything that is wanted."

The third category, the **Manipulative Help-Rejecter,** has an insatiable need for emotional support, like the Dependent Clinger and Entitled Demander. This third group is neither grateful nor aggressive, but rather feels that no therapeutic maneuver will help them. These are the patients for whom nothing works. These are the patients who return with a new complaint when one symptom is apparently relieved. As Groves so aptly states: "What is sought is an undivorceable marriage with an inexhaustible caregiver. Such patients seem to use their symptoms as an admission ticket to a relationship that cannot be sundered so long as symptoms exist."

The **Self-Destructive Denier** finds his "main pleasure in furiously defeating the physician's attempts to preserve his life." This is the patient who, with advancing cirrhosis, continues to drink. Or it is the patient who, having suffered amputations of his arms and legs because of circulatory problems caused by cigarette smoking, still balances a cigarette on his shoulder to take a few drags, or witness his roommate who smokes a cigarette through his tracheostomy. These patients are in a slow dance with death, and are extremely difficult to care for (and care about). Of the four character types, the Self-Destructive Denier is the most uncommon. The Manipulative Help-Rejecter is the most frequently encountered by physicians, but all four at once are uncommon in any practice. What is most common is a human being with a tendency for all these failings. I will tell you about one such human being.

A story . . . . several years ago, on his way through town one bright summer day, a tourist became ill. He experienced severe pain and burning in his leg while stopped at a filling station. The attendant directed him to our hospital. My partners and I, for reasons which will become clear later, all met him when he arrived in the emergency room. He had a severe infection of his lower leg together with clotting of one of the major veins in his leg, an altogether serious condition and one for which he had to be hospitalized. Flexing his muscles, he initially became an "Entitled Demander," aggressively attempting to direct his own care and demanding continual attention. He then abruptly shifted to the role of the "Dependent Clinger," requesting repeated reassurance that he would get well, that we would be able to treat his condition, and that despite being in this small rural hospital in a small backwater town, his care would be optimal. Using a brand of emotional blackmail to exact the kind of care he was demanding, he was effusive in his gratitude before we had really done anything for him. He was a desperate man, this Professor of Medicine and Chairman of his Department at a major university medical school. A famous, powerful man, he found himself in a small New England town where only the three of us knew who he really was.

We found a way around him. We told him, with faces as straight as we could manage, that we had only leeches and bloodsuckers to work with, but *for him* we would try to fly in some penicillin from Boston. *For him,* we would consider thinning his blood to deal with the inflammation in his veins, rather than simply removing his leg by amputation. *For him* we would use aspirin for his fever rather than buckets of cold water. *For him ...,* and we went on until we were all laughing, and his anxiety was diffused.

HOW TO BE A GOOD PATIENT

Recognizing that none of us as patients are *that* bad, nevertheless how can we be good patients?

We can be as honest as is humanly possible about our medical histories, honest about our own behavior and habits good and bad, and honest about our own symptoms as serious as they may be and however much we wish to deny them. Realizing that we are human beings, we can realize that our doctor is a human being as well. That will help. When a patient acknowledges that a doctor is not inexhaustible and needs to take a break, needs to see his family, needs to get some sleep, needs to take a walk in the woods with the dog, needs to read to his children, needs to be permitted to have a bad day — when a patient can acknowledge that a doctor has these needs — that patient *cares* for his doctor.

When I think of my favorite patients, what do I think of? I *enjoy* seeing them come in. They have interests that they've shared with me, are aware of my interests as well, and love to talk to me about both. They are honest about how they feel. If they are not well, they tell me so, rather than lie to me to please me and to make me think that everything is fine and that my therapy is just perfect, thank you, so that I will be pleased and not put out. If there are social conditions extraneous to their medical problems — a divorce, a sick child, a terminally ill parent — they will trust me to tell me about these things. If they do not need to see me as often, they will tell me so. And if they need to see me more often, they will ask for that as well. If there is something I am not giving them, they will tell me. And if there is something I am giving them, they thank me for it. From these patients there is the occasional postcard from Florida, usually a Christmas card, and sometimes even a jar of freezer jam. Those are the special treasures of country medicine that nothing can take away.

COMPLYING WITH MEDICAL ADVICE

Patients do not comply with medical advice because they either do not understand the instructions; they do not follow therapeutic recommendations because of side effects, discomfort or difficult behavioral patterns; or they do not comply because of denial. If patients do not understand the instructions for a certain therapy, the physician has not adequately explained it. If patients stop taking medicines or stop following therapy because of untoward side effects or discomfort, it is because the physician has not warned the patient of these side effects and has not advised the patient of a proper course of action should these side effects occur. If the patient does not comply because of substantial denial, it is because the physician has not anticipated that denial or has not broken through it. **Almost always, patient noncompliance is the responsibility of the physician.**

The number of patients who do not comply with their physicians' recommendations is hard to measure, but a reasonable estimate is that 50 percent of patients do not adhere to prescribed medical recommendations. Patients may fail to comply because they do not understand instructions or because they experience side effects. Typical are the following patients: One patient, on blood pressure medication, assumes that a short course of blood pressure medication, a month or two, will "cure" the condition. His doctor has not taught him otherwise. The patient assumes that hypertension, like pneumonia, can be cured with a short course of medication. This patient has no awareness that blood pressure medication must be taken for life. A second patient, also on blood pressure medication, and typically male in this example, experiences side effects from the medication — most commonly, impotence. Because he's embarrassed and because he has not been forewarned, he avoids both medication and physician.

Behavioral patterns are difficult for any of us to change. The smoker, the habitual drinker, the overeater, all have difficulty with compliance and understandably so. The denier has a behavioral problem, is more typically male, and denies or "forgets" the existence of his serious heart condition. He shovels snow or "tests his heart" with a jog.

If noncompliance is primarily the *doctor's* fault, what can a *patient* do about it? Communication is the key, the solution really to almost every troubled relationship. You should always understand in what manner and for how long medication should be taken. The more complicated the medical regimen, the more detailed the instructions need to be. If necessary, ask for and get printed instructions. Understand and ask about side effects, cost, and the consequences of not following the recommended regimen. Call your doctor's office if you are confused. Call your doctor's office if you have questions. Yes, you like your doctor, you respect his privacy, you understand how busy he is. But we've gone through the process of picking the right doctor for you, the kind of doctor who will have mechanisms in place in his or her office to deal with your calls and questions. Try to recognize your own tendency to deny illness. And remember the "grim reaper." Remember that your life is at stake. And finally, develop the art of communicating with your doctor.

TALKING WITH YOUR DOCTOR

There are two impediments to effective doctor-patient communication. Physicians fail to see themselves as patients see their physicians. And secondly, doctors and patients have different ideas of why disease occurs.

Let's first consider the image of a physician. A physician, in the eyes of a patient, has a profound amount of authority and power. You, as a patient, feel quite inferior. You are reluctant to interrupt, contradict, correct, or clarify — reluctant to complain or to admit that a certain drug just doesn't work. You pick up signals, nonverbal cues, that the doctor is in a hurry or is disinterested, or preoccupied. You don't want to bother him or burden him. And besides, the intimacy of the encounter causes you to forget. You have even forgotten your list. But if you can develop some rapport, some camaraderie with your physician and if you can allow him to do the same, this discomfort will lessen.

An example . . . . There are many patients who have come to me with fishing stories. On and on they go about the salmon they lost with its last leap, about the brook trout they hooked on that smallest of flies. And then there is that special effort, that pause, the glance at me, and the question: "Do you fish?" And we are off and running.

That sense of commonality will serve as a touchstone for you to break the ice for both of you in subsequent appointments. And whatever that touchstone is, whether it is books or art or music, it will make your doctor human and it will make you more than simply "a patient."

I must tell you another story. For many years in my practice I was impressed by the many and varied interests my patients had, interests I shared with them. I found myself talking about astronomy with one or gardening with another, about literature with this patient and fly-fishing with the next. It took me many years, but it finally dawned on me. These people were focusing on *my* interests. They came back often only once a year, but at the same time of year, year after year. They had bothered to learn about me, — that for me spring meant fly-fishing; summer, gardening and grapevines; fall, mushroom hunting; and winter, cross-country skiing under the stars. And those threads of commonality — those things shared — have made my practice a rich tapestry indeed. Most of these people have ceased to be merely patients. They have become my friends.

WHY DID IT HAPPEN TO ME?

Patients often think of disease as something visited upon them because of something they have done, because of some breach of behavior, because of a certain lifestyle adopted, because of the aging process itself, or because of something they deserve. In their theory of disease, guilt may predominate. These notions of causality are true only a small proportion of the time. Physicians at the same time, when hearing the list of complaints, think in terms of physiology, diet, infection, or metabolism gone awry. When people talk on two different wavelengths, how well do they communicate? If a doctor can remind himself of how patients think about disease and mollify the guilt, that will greatly help communication. And if a patient can understand more about her body, about disease processes, and about accepted theories of disease, that too will lead to a meeting of minds.

There are certain key points in giving a history to a doctor (Table 3-1). Beyond these, here are a few suggestions:

Talk about your most important complaint first, and make it clear to the doctor that that complaint is paramount. If you don't, you may never get to that complaint, or your doctor may misinterpret your priorities. He may assume your chest pain is no more

TABLE 3–1   Necessary Information in Giving a Medical History

1. On what date did the complaint start? How long did it last? How often did it come? Did it come at any particular time of day? What other symptoms occurred when it did come? If it was pain or discomfort, was it steady when it did come or did it fluctuate or come spasmodically? Did it ever occur in the past?

2. How would you characterize the complaint in terms of location on the body, tendency to travel to other parts of the body, and comparison with known sensations, such as a prickly sensation, or a numbness, or a falling asleep of an extremity, etc.

3. How would you characterize the severity of the complaint? Was it the worst headache you ever had?

4. What maneuver made the symptom worse? Or better?

5. What other factors were associated with your complaint (e.g., severe abdominal cramping associated with diarrhea)?

6. Describe in detail the worst episode you experienced.

7. What do you think the complaint represents in terms of a diagnosis? What are you afraid it *might* represent (What do you need to be reassured about)?

important to you than your back pain. Convey as honestly as you can how serious *you* think the problem might be. It is very helpful to your doctor if you tell him that this most recent headache, for example, was the most excruciating headache you have ever experienced. That kind of statement speaks volumes to a doctor. If you say that the chest pain you got while splitting wood sent a wave of terror over you, that is more helpful to the physician than all the testing in the world. Telling your doctor what you think the cause of the problem might be is an important way of revealing your own thought processes, your own ideas of causality of disease. It gets you both on the same wavelength. When a fifty-year-old woman tells me "I've got this little breast lump but I

think it's because I was carrying my grandson around,"
I immediately understand several things from this. She
is worried about a breast lump but doesn't want to
admit it. She may be exercising a great deal of denial,
wanting to believe that her problem is trivial. She trusts
me enough to tell me and is hoping I will look into it, yet
a part of her doesn't want me to. And she might think
that breast trauma is the cause of breast cancer.

Rx————————————————————————————

Quick Tips to a Complete Medical History

- Make some detailed notes before your appointment.
- Detail your present complaint using Table 3-1.
- Collect the dates and reasons for your past surgeries.
- List your past hospitalizations.
- Record the dates of your past immunizations.
- Make a list of your present medications.
- List your allergies.
- Record your smoking and drinking habits (be honest!).
- List a detailed family history (very important): your
  parents' ages, or ages at death and reasons for death;
  significant illnesses that seem to run in the families; the
  ages and health status of your siblings.
- Give a brief sketch of your social history (a key to
  rapport and helpful to a doctor considering certain
  diseases): place of birth, schooling, marriage, children,
  occupation.

WHAT PILLS ARE YOU TAKING?

The use of medication is extremely important in giving
a medical history to your doctor. Countless hours are
wasted and millions of dollars spent testing because a
patient forgets to tell the doctor, or the doctor forgets to
ask, whether certain medications or drugs might have
caused a given symptom. For example, many heart
patients mistakenly believe that nitroglycerin is an
analgesic or pain reliever, similar to aspirin, codeine, or
morphine. (Nitroglycerin actually works in another
way, to be discussed in Chapter Nine). Heart patients

may take nitroglycerin for a headache. The nitroglycerin can drop the blood pressure to very low levels, causing the headache to worsen, causing the heart to beat rapidly, causing the patient to sweat profusely, and giving the patient a sense of shock or a fear of brain hemorrhage. What has happened here? The patient took the nitroglycerin for the wrong reason. The nitroglycerin caused all of the subsequent symptoms. And because the doctor is unaware that the nitroglycerin started this whole business, he may embark on expensive testing, wasting time and money. It is most helpful to me in caring for a patient when the patient brings in the medicine bottles or a detailed list of medications and tells me how he takes them.

Finally, as in all relationships, honesty is still the best policy. The most honest statement I ever had from a patient was this: "Look Doc, I want you to keep me alive on *my* terms." Here is a patient with little self-control who realizes it, who is concerned about his health, and who is aware of the health problems his habits are causing. But most importantly, he has defined in a very helpful way the basis of our relationship. Honesty in a doctor-patient relationship implies trust, and trust, in turn, implies absolute confidence. The physician you have chosen will treat confidence in a patient-doctor relationship as a priest treats the confessional. The physician is not in the business of making moral judgments. If your doctor is to take proper care of you, he or she should know about excessive drinking, abuse of drugs, marital discord, impulsive abuse, the secret affair. And none of this need go in your medical record. Request that of your doctor. Demand it, if you must. These days, almost anyone with a good lawyer can get his hands on your medical record. That is a sad fact of "modern" American medicine.

You have found a well-trained doctor and you have decided that he or she is a good doctor as well. You will work on rapport and a sense of how to communicate. How often should you have a checkup? What should you have checked up? Under what risks do you live? What should you worry about, and what should be changed in your lifestyle? What should be altered in your environment? In your diet? These are subjects for the next chapter.

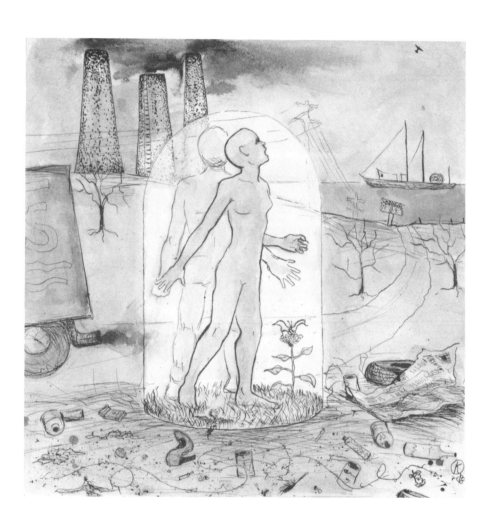

4

A Wise Man's Part: Preventative Medicine

"It is a wise man's part rather to avoid sickness than to wish for medicines."

*Sir Thomas More
(1478-1535)*

The healthiest person in America is a woman who lives on a farm with her husband, is happily married, and has a graduate degree. Her family is noted for its remarkable longevity and her brothers and sisters all enjoy excellent health. As a part-time farmer, she enjoys heavy physical labor and, beyond that, exercises for a half hour five times a week. She has a stress-free life, feels happy most of the time, and is envied by her friends for her easygoing manner. Not being a physician, she gets plenty of sleep. She has never smoked, drinks only occasionally, and takes no medicines or vitamins. She is very careful about her diet, maintains her ideal weight, eats fish three or four times a week, and never eats red meats, preferring chicken (which of course she raises herself). Her diet, however, is primarily of fruits and vegetables, almost all home-grown, and she abhors the use of pesticides and herbicides.

She has had the air in her home and her drinking water tested for radon, she always wears a seatbelt and has had a seatbelt and a rollbar installed on her tractor. She avoids chainsaws, motorcycles, and handguns. She gets a checkup once a year, has mammograms every other year, and performs monthly breast self-examination. Her idea is to avoid disease, not to look for a pill. An ounce of prevention . . . .

TAKING RISKS

None of us lives the perfect life. We all take risks, perceive risks differently one from the other, and try to do the best we can, most of the time.

- How can you evaluate risk?
- What actions vis-a-vis risk taking are appropriate?
- Are diet drinks more risky than Hudson River water?
- Do you really need to raise your own meat?
- How risky is it to live near a nuclear reactor? Or to live in Los Angeles? Or to fly on a commercial airline?

- Should you raise your children in the city or in the country?

The answers are complicated. There are facts and there are points of view. The facts, as best as they can be obtained, are immutable. Points of view are not; they are subject to lobbyists, big business, consumerism, politics, profit-and-loss, litigation, and most of all, the media. Attitudes toward the regulation of the hazards of Valium, the most frequently prescribed minor tranquilizer, are just as strong as attitudes toward the regulation of the burning of coal and other fossil fuels. Why is this? Could it have anything to do with jobs, competitive industries, or media hype? Who lobbies for Earth's atmosphere as well as is done so energetically for pharmaceutical companies? What appears to be true on television may not always be so. Statistics are a tricky thing to discuss, and even more difficult to comprehend.

I want to present to you a way to evaluate risk distinct from your perception of risk. Risk and perception of risk are two very different things. We *perceive* it to be more risky to fly in a commercial airline than to drive a car on the Interstate. But the automobile is far more risky than the commercial airliner. Keep in mind that we are talking about *relative* risks, rather than *absolute* risk. Absolute risk is extremely difficult to measure — sometimes it is impossible to measure. To say it another way: It is more hazardous to drive your car on a per mile basis than to fly Delta. And it is impossible to predict what the absolute risk of your motor trip may be, although you can reduce your relative risks by attending to speed, road conditions, substance abuse while driving, and the state of repair of your brakes and tires. Or to use another example: You are not in danger of developing cancer from exposure to chromium or coal-burning emissions, unless you live just downwind. Or consider the relative risks surrounding the asbestos controversy. Careless removal of asbestos can be a far greater risk than asbestos left in place in good repair.

THE RELATIVE RISKS OF LIFE

The simple test in Table 4-1 can give you a feeling for the relative importance of potential hazards we encounter. First, do the exercise in Table 4-1, but *do not bet on your score and cancel your life insurance policy!* This exercise illustrates the importance of not smoking, of controlling your weight, of getting regular exercise, and of avoiding or controlling stress. Some points in the test are debatable; some statisticians quarrel with the idea of less risk with rural life, and certainly a stressful, unhappy marriage can hardly be thought to be better than life alone. The test does not consider certain occupations (such as coal mining or law enforcement), nor does it consider possible exposure to radon and other cancer-causing pollutants. But the test does give you an idea of priorities; it makes little sense to uproot your family and move to the farm for your own health's sake if you smoke cigarettes and are significantly overweight.

Table 4-2 looks at risks in a slightly different way. It shows the cost in life expectancy for certain health hazards — quite revealing when we consider our preoccupation with nuclear accidents and artificial sweeteners as compared to our cavalier attitudes towards smoking and obesity. The absolute numbers of days lost is less important than the relative ranking of risk.

Ask yourself the question: How do I perceive the difference in risk between the taking of birth control pills and the problem of being 30 percent overweight? Generally, women perceive birth control pills to be a far greater danger than obesity. Table 4-2 shows just how much more hazardous obesity is than oral contraception.

CARCINOGENS: CANCER-CAUSING AGENTS

Some physical, chemical, and biologic agents are known to cause cancer in humans. These agents have been labeled **human carcinogens.** Other agents, known to cause cancers in laboratory animals, but not linked to human cancers, are considered *possible* human carcinogens. Ultraviolet rays from the sun, for example, are known human carcinogens, causing skin cancers.

TABLE 4–1 Calculating Your Life Expectancy

Start with the number 72.

Personal Facts	*Life-Style Status*
If you are male, *subtract 3.*	If you work behind a desk, *subtract 3.*
If you are female, *add 4.*	If your work requires regular, heavy
If you live in a city over two million,	physical labor, *add 3.*
subtract 2.	If you exercise strenuously five times a
If you live in a town under 10,000 or	week for 1/2 hour or more, *add 4.*
on a farm, *add 2.*	Two or three times a week, *add 2.*
If any grandparent lived to 85, *add 2.*	If you sleep more than ten hours each
If all four grandparents lived to 80,	night, *subtract 4.*
add 6.	If you are aggressive, intense, easily
If either parent died of a stroke or	angered, *subtract 3.*
heart attack before 50, *subtract 4.*	If you are easygoing and relaxed,
If any immediate family member	*add 3.*
under 50 has had cancer or a heart	If happy, *add 1;* if unhappy,
condition or diabetes since	*subtract 2.*
childhood, *subtract 3.*	If you've had a speeding ticket in the
If you earn over $50,000 a year,	past year, *subtract 1.*
subtract 2.	If you smoke more than two packs of
If you finished college, *add 1.*	cigarettes per day, *subtract 8;* one to
If you have a graduate or professional	two packs, *subtract 6;* one-half to
degree, *add 2.*	one, *subtract 3.*
If you are 65 or over and still work,	If you regularly drink 1 1/2 ounces of
add 3.	liquor a day or the equivalent,
If you live with a spouse or friend,	*subtract 1.*
add 5.	If you are overweight by 50 pounds or
If you live alone, *subtract 1 for every*	more, *subtract 8;* 30 to 50 pounds,
ten years alone since age 25.	*subtract 4;* 10 to 30 pounds,
	subtract 2.
	If you are a man over 40 and have
	annual checkups, *add 2.* If you are a
	woman and see a gynecologist once
	a year, *add 2.*

Age adjustment: For between 30 and 40, *add 2.* Between 40 and 50, *add 3.* Between 50 and 70, *add 4.* If you are over 70, *add 5.*

National average lifespans: 70.5 years for white males, 65.3 years for all other males; 78.1 years for white females, 74 years for all other females.

Source: From *Lifegain,* by Robert F. Allen, PhD., with Shirley Linde, Appleton Books, Prentice-Hall, Inc. Reprinted with permission.

TABLE 4-2   The Risks of Life

Risk Factor	Cost in Life Expectancy*
Unmarried male	3,500 days
Male cigarette smoker	2,250 days
Heart disease	2,100 days
30% overweight	1,300 days
Coal miner	1,100 days
Serving in the Army in Viet Nam	400 days
Motor vehicle accident	207 days
Average amount of alcohol intake	130 days
Home accident	95 days
Coffee drinker	6 days
Oral contraceptive user	5 days
Diet drink consumer	2 days
Nuclear accident	2 days

*Source: Derived from life insurance acturial tables on life expectancy and insurability.

Radiation is another such physical carcinogen. Certain viruses — **biologic carcinogens** — and a whole host of chemical agents have also been shown to produce cancers in both laboratory animals and in humans.

Turn now to Table 4-3, but not before memorizing a key statement: **The use of tobacco accounts for more cancers among Americans than all other known carcinogens combined; one quarter of all cancer deaths in the United States can be attributed to the use of tobacco. Look at a few numbers: In a study of Americans from twenty-five states over twelve years, out of a population of one million smokers, 150,000 of those smokers died of cancer.**

We come to an important concept: risk juxtaposed against the *perception* of risk. We may realize the dangers of cigarette smoking and choose not to smoke ourselves, but are more concerned about government control of pesticide use than we are about tobacco subsidies. Think about it. The distortions that perceived

TABLE 4–3   The Relative Risks of Possible
Carcinogens

Possible Hazard (HERP%)	Daily Human Exposure	Carcinogen Contained
Environmental Pollutants		
0.001	Tap water, 1 liter	Chloroform
0.004	Contaminated well water, 1 liter	Trichloroethylene
0.008	Swimming pool, 1 hour	Chloroform
0.6	Conventional home air, 14 hours per day	Formaldehyde
2.1	Mobile home air, 14 hours per day	Formaldehyde
Pesticides and Other Residues		
0.0002	PCBs, daily dietary intake	PCBs
0.0004	EDBs, daily dietary intake (from grains)	Ethylene dibromide
Natural Pesticides and Dietary Toxins		
0.003	Bacon, cooked	Nitrosamines
0.03	Comfrey herb tea, 1 cup	Symphytine
0.03	Peanut butter, 1 sandwich	Aflatoxins
0.07	Brown mustards, 5 grams	Isothiocyanates
0.1	Basil, 1 gram of a dried leaf	Estragole
0.1	One raw mushroom, 15 grams	Hydrazines
2.8	Beer, 12 ounces	Ethyl alcohol
4.7	Wine, 4 ounces	Ethyl alcohol
Food Additives		
0.06	Diet cola, 12 ounces	Saccharin
Drugs (Average Dose)		
5.6	Metronidazole	Metronidazole, 2000 mg
14	Isoniazid	Isoniazid, 300 mg
16	Phenobarbital	Phenobarbital, 60 mg
17	Clofibrate	Clofibrate, 2000 mg

(*continues*)

TABLE 4–3 (continued)

Possible Hazard (HERP%)	*Daily Human Exposure*	*Carcinogen Contained*
	Occupational Exposure	
5.8	Formaldehyde, workers' average	Formaldehyde
140	EDBs, workers' daily intake (high exposure)	Ethylene dibromide

Source: "Ranking Possible Carcinogenic Hazards," Bruce N. Ames, *et al.,* Vol. 236, pp. 271-280, Table 1, April 17, 1987, *Science*. Reprinted with permission.

risk can generate result in almost a national schizophrenia. We pay taxes for the Food and Drug Administration and yet fund the tobacco industry. We establish the Environmental Protection Agency and do nothing about acid rain.

Table 4-3 is a list of *possible* human carcinogens, *known* to be *rodent* carcinogens, listed in groups and in order of increasing risk according to possible hazard. The numbers at the left, the HERP percentages, are, for our purposes, important only for relative comparisons. They relate *H*uman *E*xposure to *R*odent *P*otency. In other words, it is the relationship between human susceptibility and testing on rodents. The percentages will give you an appreciation for the relative importance of things. Table 4-3 shows the potential relative risks of several rodent carcinogens based on *daily* human exposure. Certain comparisons are interesting. Drinking contaminated well water has less possible hazard in terms of potential for cancer than does drinking diet cola sweetened with saccharin. The aflatoxins found in peanut butter are far more potentially hazardous than the average American's dietary intake of certain pesticides. And *neither* are of the same magnitude as the risk from tobacco. You would need to breathe Los Angeles smog for a year or more to breathe the same amount of pollutants that a two-packs-a-day smoker gets in a day.

A comparison of commonplace risks can be seen in

Table 4-4. This list gives relative comparisons of cigarette smoking (and peanut butter) to both carcinogens and noncancer-causing hazards. The table tells us, doesn't it, how penny-wise, pound-foolish we can be.

A story about a woman of precaution . . . . Once upon a time there was a woman with a list. And on this list were the risks of everything, all jotted down in percentages and days and life expectancy and 0.2 percent this and seventy more days of that and so on and so on. She was very good at this and patterned her day after her list so that she could eliminate all hazards. She never smoked and she avoided smoke-filled rooms. If she wished to visit a city, she would avoid those known especially to be smog-laden and therefore containing atmospheres filled with carcinogens. She avoided the nitrites in processed meats, the cholesterol in dairy products, and the merest possibility of car-

TABLE 4–4   Some Commonplace Hazards in Order of *Decreasing* Risk

1. Cigarette smoking, one pack per day
2. All cancers
3. Mountaineering (mountaineers)
4. Motor vehicle accidents (total)
5. Policeman killed in line of duty
6. Air pollution, eastern United States
7. Home accidents
8. Frequent flying businessman
9. Motor vehicle accident (pedestrians only)
10. Sea-level background radiation (except radon)
11. Alcohol, light drinker
12. Four tablespoons of peanut butter per day
13. Electrocution
14. Drinking water with EPA limit of chloroform
15. Drinking water with EPA limit of trichloroethylene

Source: "Perception of Risk," Paul Slovic, Vol. 236, pp. 280-285, Table 1, Figures 1, 2, 3, and 4, April 17, 1987, *Science*. Reprinted with permission.

cinogens in irradiated food. She would not allow foreign substances to enter her body: She never took birth control pills, never smoked, abhorred pills in general, and preferred to take her vitamins through a well-balanced diet. She grew her own vegetables, because you never know. Ever careful about additives, she purchased her meat using utmost scrutiny, and she scorned diet drinks and processed foods in general.

She campaigned against the dangers of radiation. She marched for a nuclear-free world, helped her neighbors test for radon, and avoided radiation of any sort. This included radiation from diagnostic X-rays such as mammograms. At age forty-nine, and healthy in all other respects, she died of breast cancer.

THE HAZARDS OF RADIATION

An important indoor air pollutant receiving a lot of press these days is the radioactive gas called *radon*. The Northeast in general, and Maine in particular with its granite ledges, holds large veins of low-level radioactive granite. The radioactive substances in the granite emit a radioactive gas called radon. This gas gets dissolved in the ground water and is inhaled in shower stalls during long showers. Radon also seeps in from granite ledges through foundations into the basements of houses, allowing for exposure in another way. Radon's radioactive decay products are cancer-causing.

Diagnostic X-rays are also a source of radiation, although the risk is very small. Yet because of society's perception of risk, it often takes a court order to get a person to accept a diagnostic X-ray, although anyone would risk flying to Disneyland. There are many other sources of radiation as well. These radiation sources can be carcinogenic; some are listed in Table 4-5, which shows a relative comparison of radiation risks, including the risk from radon exposure. Note that the risk of living very near to a nuclear power plant is extremely small. But we musn't forget Chernobyl.

These are some of the *facts* about health risks. In later chapters we will examine in more detail some of these health risks (or as physicians refer to them, "risk factors") such as diet, obesity, lack of exercise, alcohol

TABLE 4–5 Comparison of Some Common Radiation Risks

Physical Agent	Dose (mrem*/ year)	Cancers if all U.S. population were exposed
Medical X-rays	40	1100
Radon gas	500	13,500
Potassium in own body	30	1000
Cosmic radiation at sea level	40	1100
Cosmic radiation at Denver	65	1800
Radiation exposure to average resident near Chernobyl in the first year	5000	Not relevant
Cosmic radiation during one transcontinental round trip by air	5	135
Average radiation within 20 miles of a nuclear power plant	0.02	>1

*mrem=millirem, a unit of measurement for radiation.
Source: "Risk Assessment and Comparisons: An Introduction," R. Wilson and E. A. C. Crouch, Vol. 236, pp. 267-270, April 17, 1987, *Science*. Reprinted with permission.

and tobacco. And we will in a moment consider one maneuver that can improve your chances of meeting your grandchildren: *the checkup*. Before we do, let us consider how we perceive risk.

PERCEPTION OF HEALTH RISKS

How we perceive risk is important when making decisions about taking care of ourselves. We perceive risks differently depending upon who we are, how much we believe the media, and how much denial we can exercise with regard to poor personal habits. In short, most of us believe what we want to believe.

Table 4-6 shows how differently different groups of people think about risk. Thirty activities and technologies are ranked according to *perceived* risk. Four

TABLE 4–6 Perceived Risk for 30 Activities and Technologies

Activity or Technology	Ranking*			
	League of Women Voters	College Students	Active Club Members	Experts
Nuclear power	1	1	8	20
Motor vehicles	2	5	3	1
Handguns	3	2	1	4
Smoking	4	3	4	2
Motorcycles	5	6	2	6
Alcoholic beverages	6	7	5	3
General (private) aviation	7	15	11	12
Police work	8	8	7	17
Pesticides	9	4	15	8
Surgery	10	11	9	5
Fire fighting	11	10	6	18
Large construction	12	14	13	13
Hunting	13	18	10	23
Spray cans	14	13	23	26
Mountain climbing	15	22	12	29
Bicycles	16	24	14	15
Commercial aviation	17	16	18	16
Electric power (non-nuclear)	18	19	19	9
Swimming	19	30	17	10
Contraceptives	20	9	22	11
Skiing	21	25	16	30
X-rays	22	17	24	7
High school and college football	23	26	21	27
Railroads	24	23	20	19
Food preservatives	25	12	28	14
Food coloring	26	20	30	21
Power mowers	27	28	25	28
Prescription antibiotics	28	21	26	24
Home appliances	29	27	27	22
Vaccinations	30	29	29	25

*A rank of 1 represents the most risky activity or technology.

Source: "Perception of Risk," Paul Slovic, Vol. 236, pp. 280-285, Table 1, April 17, 1987, *Science*. Reprinted with permission.

groups of people — The League of Women Voters, college students, active club members, and experts — ranked the activities or technologies from 1 to 30, with 1 representing the most risky activity or technology. Rather than think about who is correct, get a sense for how perceptions may differ; then ask yourself why. Experts tend to judge risk according to annual fatality whereas lay people judge risk more in terms of catastrophic potential or threat to future generations. Table 4-6 represents how different groups think about risk. Table 4-4 gives us, in simplified fashion, *the facts*.

Maine was selected as a potential dump site for radioactive waste. The local media sprang into action. Hardly an hour went by that we didn't see someone on television condemning this silly idea or read something in the newspapers opposing Maine as a radioactive dump site. We had signs in our windows, signs on the front lawn, signs on our bumpers. We met, agitated, wrote letters, yelled, and screamed until the trucks filled with waste turned back. We perceived the risk, to ourselves and to future generations, correctly to be great, and we did something about it. Our *perception* of the risk had been heightened. The media had helped us with that perception, and the media, in turn, had acted in part because of the distress of realtors, landowners, and businessmen.

We have another problem, in Maine and elsewhere, whose risks are not as well perceived. Any teenage boy in a pickup can buy a six-pack of beer almost as easily as he can purchase a package of gum. It is a way of life here in Maine. Some think it is their *right* not to wear their seatbelts, their *right* to buy a six-pack and put it on the seat next to them, their *right* to drain a can of beer while they drive and throw the crushed can out the window. It is their *right* to allow their children to hit bridge abutments, wrap the truck around a telephone pole, or wipe out an entire family with a head-on crash.

But a terrible tragedy occurred in our community a few years ago to change that perception of risk, the risk of drunk-driving. On graduation night several years ago six drunken teenagers missed a bridge entirely and

drove over a banking, into a river. All six high school
graduates drowned. Our emergency room that evening
was filled with weeping parents, hysterical classmates,
stricken law enforcement officers and horrified ambulance technicians. Out of this pathos came the idea for
"Project Graduation," and out of Project Graduation
came, finally, media support opposing drunk-driving,
promoting instead alternate forms of celebration on
graduation night. The idea for Project Graduation has
spread from Maine, to the rest of New England, and to
the entire nation. We have now at least one night a year
when the perception of the risk of drunk-driving is
heightened. It's a wonderful beginning.

THE CHECKUP The healthiest person in America gets an annual
physical examination. Is this an informed decision on
her part, or is she lining some doctor's pocket? Is *not*
getting an annual checkup a health risk in itself? This
is a big area of controversy in medicine. Many experts
believe periodic physical examinations are essential.
Others feel just the opposite. They cost money, and
insurance companies don't want to pay for them.
Neither does the federal government; it has aircraft
carriers to worry about. Sad but true, many insurance
companies refuse to pay for screening tests for cancer
on healthy individuals, yet will pay thousands of
dollars caring for the cancer patient whose chance for
early diagnosis has been missed.

What is a reasonable approach to the checkup?
What should you expect to have looked at and which
diagnostic tests should you expect to have performed?
Here's what I tell my patients:

- If you are *male* and between the ages of twenty and
  forty years, get a physical examination every five
  years. Between age forty and fifty, get one every
  year or every other year, depending upon your
  state of health. After age fifty, get a physical
  examination annually.
- Women, between twenty and forty years of age,

should have an *annual* breast examination and a pelvic examination with a Pap smear. Get a *complete* physical examination every five years. Continue annual breast and pelvic examinations after age forty for the rest of your life but get a complete physical examination every one to two years, depending upon your health status. After age fifty, get a physical examination done annually.

- Women should perform *monthly* breast self-examination (see Chapter Ten) after age twenty. Similarly, men should perform a monthly self-examination for testicular cancer.
- Women should get an annual breast X-ray examination done after age forty unless risk factors dictate otherwise (see Chapter Ten).
- Periodic tests for hypertension, blood cholesterol, anemia, and a test for occult blood in the stool should be done. The interval of such testing will depend upon age, family history, and other risk factors as discussed in subsequent chapters.
- A baseline electrocardiogram is an essential part of your medical record after the age of forty.
- Examination of the rectum and lower colon by the use of a flexible fiberoptic tube (*flexible sigmoidoscopy*) should be performed every three to five years after the age of fifty (more on this in Chapter Ten).
- Certain immunizations are important for adults: Every adult should have a tetanus-diphtheria booster every ten years. Influenza vaccine should be given to all patients over the age of sixty and to younger patients who are at high risk because of coexisting chronic diseases such as heart disease, lung diseases, diabetes, kidney disease, or cancer. All nonpregnant women of childbearing age should have a vaccination against German measles (rubella). High risk patients (those listed for whom the flu vaccine is indicated), especially those with lung disease and especially those who have had a spleen removed, should be vaccinated against a specific kind of pneumonia (Pneumovax).

Does it matter whether you see the *same* physician for each checkup? Is it crucial to your health to have your own personal physician? That depends on how you view medicine — how much you view medicine as science, and how much as art. Those who are about the business of managing health care — busily marketing "health care products" — want you to believe that medicine is all science, a packaged product to be sold off the shelf. But a great deal of art goes into the practice of medicine. That is something I have learned from twenty years in practice. I have found that patients need to trust me before they will tell me things — not a startling discovery, certainly. Such trust rarely develops in one visit to the doctor's office.

Another story . . . . Several years ago I was employed as a physician in a grand Health Maintenance Organization called the United States Army. They permitted me to see patients much as I might see them in a private office.

One day the wife of an Army captain came to see me. She was thirty years old, had three small children, and complained of extreme fatigue all out of proportion to the malaise commonly experienced by mothers of small children. She could barely keep her eyes open during the day, could barely function, and was worried about her abilities to care for her children. This lethargy had been going on for months. Her husband had finally convinced her to see a physician about it.

Her medical history, in all other respects, was unremarkable. She had never been hospitalized, nor had she ever been seriously ill. She was not taking any medications. She had no family history of a similar illness — significant when considering some of the possible causes of this marked tendency to sleep (*hypersomnia,* as we call it).

She did not feel depressed. Her husband's Army career was going well, and she enjoyed her role as an officer's wife. She felt that she had no reason to be depressed. She was thin and looked chronically ill. Her physical examination, however, was quite normal. I performed a whole battery of laboratory examinations, looking for metabolic or nervous system causes of this extreme fatigue. These tests were also competely normal. I had no idea what her problem was.

After the initial examination and after the follow-up visit to review her laboratory testing, I saw her in the office once a month, mostly to get a feeling for how her problem might be progressing.

On the fourth or fifth such follow-up visit she gave me another piece of information: "There's something I haven't told you," she said. "Maybe it's important ... I don't know." She looked at me with those tired, sad eyes, bit her lower lip, and continued.

"Sometimes I feel as though there is another whole person inside me . . . another person . . . completely different ... leading a completely different life." She told me about a feeling she had of being possessed — of being taken over by another person. I began to look at her in a different light.

I then remembered an argument I had had with one of the GI's who worked in the hospital. With a snicker, he had referred to the patient as Sally. I had corrected him, telling him that her name was Evelyn. But he seemed unconvinced, and sure that he was right. Now I wondered about that confusion of names, given the additional history Evelyn was supplying.

Eventually, Evelyn's/Sally's diagnosis became clear: She had a true dual personality similar to that portrayed in *Three Faces of Eve.* By day, Evelyn was the model captain's wife. By night, Sally was a barfly known to all the GI's. As Evelyn she had a sense that Sally might exist, but needed to trust me before she could share with me those thoughts. Excellent psychiatric care helped Evelyn resolve her conflicts. Sally ceased to exist.

The moral of Evelyn's story is this:

Had she met with a different physician each visit, I wonder whether her problem would ever have been diagnosed. It mattered a great deal for her to have trust in one personal physician.

Evelyn's chief complaint had been fatigue. I had another patient complain to me of fatigue and, months later, after a considerable amount of trust had developed between us, that patient told me of his two complete families and two lives in two different towns. One life is fatiguing enough.

Fatigue is a prominent symptom of alcohol and drug abuse and of depression of many causes, but the patient rarely gives clues to the problem on the first visit.

Remember, this is a book about thinking for yourself. View with skepticism any offers of "managed" health care. Scrutinize any attempts to "provide" you with walk-in medical care. It *does* matter whether you have your own personal physician.

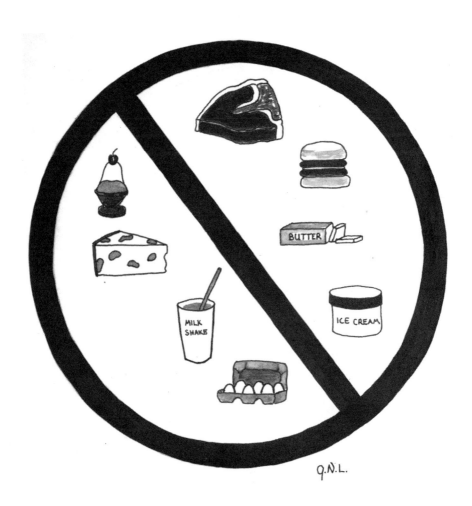

5

Sweeter Poisons: Cholesterol and Sugar

"The flesh of the mushroom Amanita virosa is reported to be delicious, especially when sauteed. Only much later, when therapy is applied too desperately and too late, do its poisons prove lethal."
J. Featherstone Privy, 1988

Once upon a time, there lived a man who worried about himself. His father had died at forty-six of a heart attack; he promised his wife and children he would not suffer the same fate. Diet and exercise, he read in the Sunday supplement, are the keys to longevity. He began to jog, barely a mile a day at first. Quickly, he learned the difference between a jogger and a runner and aspired to becoming a runner. He gave up smoking, not an easy thing to do, but it did get in the way of his running and it was, he read, another nail in the coffin of heart disease.

Weeks and months went by. His daily mileage increased, he became fit, slim, then gaunt. Now he read that those who complete a marathon will never get heart disease. Well then, he said, he would run a marathon every year. No more Sunday breakfasts of bacon and eggs with the family. No more candlelight dinners with his wife. The food was unhealthy; besides, there was no time. He began each day with a plan to get his training mileage accomplished. This day, four easy miles in the morning and then six more miles at a brisk pace after work. Tomorrow, a long run of twenty miles would be in order, and then an easy day on Friday.

Alcohol, he read, raises the "good" cholesterol. Dutifully, he had a drink each evening. Stress is bad, he read. He gave his wife the checkbook and the bills. In fact, he gave his wife more than that: He gave her total responsibility for child rearing and for running the home, which he saw as too stressful—unhealthy.

Newsbreak: One aspirin a day can prevent heart attacks! An aspirin in the morning, and a drink before dinner — certainly a healthy regimen, he figured. Oats! What about oats?! Healthy consumption of oats can lower your cholesterol! *Entire* diet books tell about it! Imagine, an entire book just about eating oats! There must be something to that, he thought. Oats for breakfast, with an aspirin, after an easy run, then a brisk middle distance run with "intervals" before the drink, before dinner, eaten quite late, after the kids are in bed. Not narcissism, certainly not, he shrugged — a healthy brand of self-absorption.

It was an open casket. He was found among the leaves at the side of the road. His friends gathered in the heavy air of the parlor and marveled at how healthy he looked at fifty-two, how fit, how trim, how dead. What had gone wrong? He had covered all of the bases. He had left no stone unturned. Or had he?

Read on and see if you can discover where our late runner tripped up.

CHOLESTEROL PROBLEMS

Shopping for a heart attack? Fill your cart with plenty of fatty foods. Excess fat in the blood is responsible for both heart disease and stroke. No one disputes that. And no one disputes the benefit of doing something about the fat in your blood. Too much fat in the blood shortens your life expectancy. It is that simple. The solution is not so simple. The solution — lifelong vigilance, lifelong dieting of a sort, lifelong medical supervision — involves a huge decision.

You need to decide how you look at medical care with respect to your lifestyle. Early diagnosis and treatment of fat and cholesterol problems does help. But you can rationalize that you cannot live forever and so ask, are the rigors of therapy really worth it? If therapy — in this case, a change in diet — is only partially successful, do you want to make the sacrifice? What does improved longevity mean to you? Are you willing to accept some degree of sacrifice in the hopes of improving comfort and well-being in the future?

A good first step is to learn about the problem. This is our topic at hand. Doctors refer to harmful blood fats — *cholesterol* and *triglycerides* — as **lipids.** These lipids, cholesterol and triglycerides, are both found in the diet and manufactured within the body. They are carried around in the bloodstream by **lipoproteins.** Things are already getting complicated. Let's simplify.

Focus on cholesterol only for a moment. Too much of it in the bloodstream and fat is deposited on the inside surfaces of blood vessels much as does the white crust found on the inside of an old pipe. If the deposits continue unchecked, more and more cholesterol is deposited until finally the blood vessel is totally blocked. When a blood clot forms in an artery, that artery can no longer supply its tissues with nutrients and oxygen. Whatever has depended upon that blood vessel will die. If the blockage, or **thrombosis,** occurs in a blood vessel supplying a portion of the brain, a stroke may occur, causing paralysis or problems of speech, or worse. If the thrombosis occurs in one of the arteries supplying heart muscle, a coronary artery, then a **coronary thrombosis** occurs and that portion of heart muscle supplied by that blood vessel dies, and a heart attack, or **myocardial infarction,** is the result.

How does the cholesterol get deposited and what can remove the deposits? Think of the lipoproteins — the substances that carry cholesterol and triglycerides around in the bloodstream — as pickup trucks. We have black pickup trucks — nasty things, obviously — and we have white pickup trucks — one can never have enough of those. The black pickup trucks are loaded with cholesterol, called *LDL cholesterol.* The white pickup trucks are also carrying cholesterol, the kind called *HDL cholesterol.* When people refer to "good cholesterol," they are talking about HDL cholesterol. When cholesterol either is manufactured in the liver or enters the body through diet, it is loaded into both white and black pickup trucks. The black pickup trucks busily dump the cholesterol onto the inside surfaces of blood vessels, where it collects and ultimately can lead to thrombosis. The white pickup trucks are in the business of taking the cholesterol out of the blood system and removing it from the body.

Immediately we can make several assumptions. If the number of pickup trucks, both black and white, is an inherited sort of thing, much like blue eyes or brown eyes, then it might be wise to choose our parents carefully. It would be preferable to inherit only a small number of black pickup trucks, together with a healthy number of white ones. And in truth, white and black pickups (lipoproteins) are governed in their amounts by modes of inheritance. Also, if there is very little cholesterol around, it really shouldn't make any difference how many pickup trucks, black or white, one has driving around in the bloodstream. This logic happens to be true: *Empty pickup trucks can do no damage.* Finally, if certain habits will increase the number of white pickup trucks, then we should certainly like to learn them.

Choosing Your Parents Carefully

Let's examine first the problem of inheritance as it relates to lipids — cholesterol and triglycerides. Your parents can and do pass on to you a great many attributes: a fantastic backhand, the ability to sing on key, and a great many black pickup trucks. In fact, it gets even worse. The ability to make incredible amounts of cholesterol within the body, or a similar ability to manufacture large amounts of triglyceride within the body, can be inherited. Similarly, the ability to remove cholesterol and triglycerides from the body, or more properly, the *inability* to do so, is also inherited. It should now be obvious to you that if you have inherited legions of black pickup trucks and very few white ones, and if you have inherited the ability to manufacture within the liver large amounts of cholesterol, it will make little difference what your diet is — you are in desperate straits. But even when in such desperate straits, therapy can help a great deal. It should also be obvious to you by now where our late runner went wrong.

If your parents don't get you in this thing, other diseases can. Certain conditions and behaviors can cause serious problems of blood lipids. Some examples: Obesity itself is related to increased blood triglycerides and cholesterol. Excessive amounts of alcohol can significantly raise triglycerides. Triglycerides can also be quite high in some diabetics. Thyroid disorders, resulting in an underactive thyroid, are commonly related to increases in blood cholesterol. Certain medications, especially cortisone-like drugs, birth control pills, and other sources of estrogen, can raise triglycerides and often cholesterol as well.

The Great American Diet is our downfall. Steak, homefries, and apple pie a la mode are red-white-and-blue. Indeed, it is un-American even to think otherwise. Ours is a society more of bad habits than bad genes. Cheeseburgers and french fries cause more cholesterol problems in Americans than all the genetic mismatches one could contrive. Oats for breakfast, with an aspirin on the side, is not going to rescue someone on the Great American Diet. Dietary change must be the core of therapy for cholesterol problems. By now, I hope that is obvious to you.

The Great American Diet
Foods Especially High in Cholesterol and Saturated Fats

Bacon double cheeseburger deluxe
Egg McMuffin
French fries (fried in animal fats)
Big Mac
Hot dog
Hot fudge sundae
Fried onion rings (fried in animal fat)
Ham and cheese sandwich
Scrambled eggs
Italian sausage sandwich
Pizza (lots of mozzarella)

Attacking a Cholesterol Problem

Media attention has made all of us aware of the importance of blood cholesterol. Even the elderly now want a cholesterol measurement, as if they might be charged twenty years off their life should they learn that their cholesterol is high.

But measurement *is* the next step: After learning about cholesterol, get a reliable blood measurement of lipids, a so-called **lipid profile.** Do *not* start improving your heart and your health with jogging, or with a diet of oats and aspirin, or with libraries of diet manuals. Start with a reliable lipid profile.

Table 5-1 contains such a profile. It is a sample laboratory test from a hospital pathology department. Section A of the profile shows actual measurements on a patient after the patient has fasted for fourteen hours. Section B interprets the tests in a certain way, which we

TABLE 5-1   Interpreting A Lipid Profile

A. Lipid Profile

Test Name	Result	Units	Reference Range
HDL cholesterol	51	mg/dl	
Total cholesterol	210	mg/dl	114-200
Triglycerides	46	mg/dl	23-158
VLDL	9	mg/dl	<40
LDL	150	mg/dl	62-185
Percent HDL cholesterol	**24**		
Cholesterol/HDL ratio	**4**		

B. Percent HDL Cholesterol

	Male	Female
Protection probable	>28	>28
Below average CHD risk	23-28	23-28
Average CHD risk	16-22	18-22
High CHD risk	7-15	9-17
CHD risk dangerous	<7	<9

C. Cholesterol/HDL Ratio

	Male	Female
Protection probable	<3.5	<3.5
Below average CHD risk	3.5-4.4	3.5-4.4
Average CHD risk	4.5-6.4	4.5-5.5
High CHD risk	6.5-13.4	5.6-10.9
CHD risk dangerous	>13.5	>11

Note: CHD = coronary heart disease.

will discuss below. Section C allows for a different interpretation of the data.

First, turn your attention to section A. The numbers give actual measurements for cholesterol, triglyceride, and the white truck/black truck lipoprotein levels. The numbers in section A that are bold face are most useful for our discussion. By taking the percentage of total cholesterol that is good cholesterol (HDL cholesterol), we get the first of the two bold numbers — in this example, 24 percent. Then, by taking a ratio of total cholesterol to HDL cholesterol, we get the second of the two bold numbers — in this case, 4. We use these two numbers to interpret for our patient the risk of developing coronary heart disease (CHD).

Section B shows us that a percent HDL cholesterol of 24 places our patient in the "below average coronary heart disease risk group," since our patient's percent HDL cholesterol falls between 23 and 28 percent. Similarly, in section C we see that a cholesterol/HDL ratio of 4 once again places our patient in the "below average coronary heart disease risk group," since 4 is between 3.5 and 4.4.

Please remember that no other risk factors are being considered when we make these predictions for our patient. We do not know whether the patient smokes, or has high blood pressure, or is significantly overweight, or has diabetes mellitus.

Further, we need to make some assumptions. A simple cholesterol measurement is not always enough information to advise the patient. For example, triglycerides can be quite high in a patient who has "normal" cholesterol. This is still a dangerous situation. Conversely, some patients, with an "abnormal" cholesterol level, can have very high levels of HDL cholesterol (good cholesterol in the white trucks) and will still have percentages and ratios placing them in the protection probable group. To repeat: A simple blood cholesterol test may not always be enough. A lipid profile is preferable.

Tragedy: Blood Cholesterol Too High

What to do? Don't panic! These days, we are talking about a treatable disorder. The idea is to recognize it early enough before significant amounts of cholesterol sludge have been dumped by the black pickup trucks. Your physician will immediately concern himself with ruling in or ruling out inheritance or certain diseases as the cause for your high blood lipids. Beyond family history, secondary causes of elevated blood lipids — diseases that may be causing the problem — can be discovered through a careful physical examination and through other testing. Your physician will look for certain skin, eye, and tendon abnormalities as a tip-off to some unknown inherited problem of lipid metabolism. He or she will test for diabetes and kidney disorders and, if indicated, disorders of the thyroid. Your physician will ask about medications; if he doesn't, remember, as stressed in Chapter Three, to bring in your list of medications or your pill bottles.

Dietary Treatment of High Blood Lipids

Let's assume your parents have been good to you in bestowing upon you normal amounts of white and black trucks. You are healthy otherwise, having no diseases other than this problem of high cholesterol. Your initial approach has to be to change your diet. That is a "wise man's part." Remember, we are not interested in pills just yet. Regardless of whether triglycerides or cholesterol is elevated, the first dietary maneuver is to lose excess weight. A vigorous, but rational, exercise program can help in this regard and can also increase HDL cholesterol — good cholesterol —at the same time.

The American Heart Association (see Bibliography) publishes several pamphlets and a cookbook employing a stepwise single diet approach to treat elevated blood lipids. This diet, in addition to encouraging loss of excess weight, restricts cholesterol and saturated fats, increases polyunsaturated fats in the diet, and, in the case of elevated triglycerides, restricts alcohol and sugar as well. These pamphlets and the cookbook will give you specific guidelines for drawing up a menu and detailed information about the amounts of cholesterol, saturated fats, and polyunsaturated fats in foods. In addition, here are some general considerations:

Fat in the diet is either **saturated** or **unsaturated.** Saturated fats in the diet can cause elevated blood cholesterol more than any other food in the diet.

Saturated fatty acids are found in most dairy products, in fatty meats, in the skin of poultry, and in the saturated fats found in nondairy creamers.

Warning: Foods can be labeled "cholesterol-free" but can still contain unhealthy amounts of saturated fatty acids (see Table 5-2).

You want to avoid both. Unsaturated fatty acids are found in safflower, sunflower, and corn oils; in margarines made from these sources; and in fish. Fish, and the oils found in fish, are especially good. EPA (Eicosapentaenoic acid) found in fish exerts a protective effect against the development of cholesterol deposits and heart disease. Societies with a high proportion of fish in their diet have been carefully studied and have been found to have remarkably low incidences of coronary disease.

I know . . . you can buy EPA capsules anywhere. Why not take those? Because we have agreed to stop looking for a pill for every problem. Taking a pill for a problem, when you don't have to, means you have given up thinking for yourself. We all need to start thinking for ourselves. Better to get a fish cookbook and start slowly incorporating fish in your diet until you have learned the pleasures of fish three or four times a week — no sauce please!

Eating foods rich in cholesterol itself can also raise blood cholesterol, although eating foods rich in saturated fatty acids is much more of a problem. High cholesterol

TABLE 5–2   Sources of Saturated Fatty Acids

Animal fat	Coconut	Palm kernel oil
Bacon fat	Coconut oil	Palm oil
Beef fat	Cream	Pork fat
Butter	Eggs	Turkey fat
Chicken fat	Ham fat	Vegetable oils (with coconut or palm oil)
Cocoa butter	Lard	Vegetable shortening

foods include egg yolks and organ meats and, to a lesser extent, dairy products and red meats.

Diet for Lowering Cholesterol

If you came to me with a cholesterol problem, had no hint of an hereditary source for this problem or of a disease causing it, here is the kind of diet I would recommend for you. My choices and biases are based as much on a knowledge of human nature as they are on absolute percentages of saturated fats and cholesterol. For example, lean beef can contain relatively little cholesterol and saturated fat, as the beef industry is now so energetically telling us. Nevertheless, when looking at a restaurant menu, our own definitions of "lean" become blurred. Let's take this diet by food groups.

Breads and Starches. This food group is pretty safe. Try to avoid breads, biscuits, and crackers made with whole milk, eggs, and saturated oils; most such commercial preparations are taboo. Creamed soups in restaurants, which are usually made with whole milk or, more commonly, cream, are also out. Canned soups are very salty and should be avoided. Note that I am assuming you also have twenty pounds to lose and wish to avoid the water retention that salt consumption can bring. Besides, a low salt diet is always a good idea. No one said this was going to be easy. One other note: Sad to say, doughnuts are not in the bread group. They are in the fat group and are taboo. No doughnuts!

Vegetables and Fruits. This is also a fairly safe group except for lovers of olives and avocados. Obviously, if you fry your vegetables or prepare them in a bechamel sauce, you are pretty adept at self-deception. About that twenty pounds you want to lose: Fruits canned in juices and sugary syrups are quite high in calories. Drain them.

Fats and Oils. Use only the unsaturated oils I mentioned above: safflower, corn, sunflower, soybean. Tub margarine is best; butter is out. Learn to live without salad dressings. Peanut butter which "contains no cholesterol!" is tricky; 50 percent of its fat is saturated fatty acid, and it is high in calories.

I have to tell you a peanut butter story . . . . I saw a patient about two years ago who had a blood cholesterol level of 376. He was thirty pounds overweight, but in all other respects, including family history, he was quite normal. I gave him the diet I am outlining here, told him to lose thirty pounds, and asked him to come back every four to six weeks so that I could keep an eye on things, weigh him in, and scold him if necessary. I didn't see him for a year. When he returned, I hardly recognized him. He was a small man — that is, short of stature —and with thirty pounds off, he looked twenty years younger. He had obviously been with the program. I asked him how he was doing.

"Doc," he said, "I was hungry all of the time until I got down to this weight . . . . I was miserable, but I did it. Now I've loosened up a bit, and I'm not hungry, but I'm not going to gain that weight back. I've done everything you said except for one thing. I couldn't give up peanut butter. I love peanut butter. I have a little bit on my toast for breakfast, take a peanut butter sandwich with me to work, and have some for supper. When you told me about the diet and what I had to do I went home and thought about it. I decided that since I was giving up so much, I would give up everything but one thing, and keep that for myself." I checked his serum cholesterol; it was 149. When I told him he grinned and said:

I guess I'm doing all right, eh Doc?

Meat Group. Avoid any and all processed meats. Processed meats include bacon, sausages, hot dogs, and luncheon meats. Avoid all organ meats, including liver. Duck and goose are taboo. Other poultry, with the skin removed before or after cooking, is fine. Have three or four servings of fish a week. Attempt meatless meals; it is actually possible to do this and survive. No eggs allowed! Certain shellfish — shrimp and lobster, for example — are high in cholesterol, but there is some debate as of this writing whether the cholesterol found in shellfish is to be avoided. To be safe, have no more than one serving of shellfish per week.

You only need about six ounces of meat per day. One-half of a chicken breast — or a chicken leg together with the thigh — is about three ounces, as is one-half a cup of fish. Remember to remove the skin from the poultry, and don't fry the fish!

You *can* remain healthy, and live a normal life, without beef. All of the nutrients found in beef are found in other foods. You do not need beef to survive.

Dairy Products. Use only skim milk. Avoid whole milk certainly and "low fat" milk of any description. Avoid cream — light, heavy, and sour. Avoid nondairy creamers; remember they are high in saturated fats. Do not eat cheese. Low-fat cheeses, *in moderation,* are acceptable. However, as students of human nature, we know that it is often easier to cut out a particular food entirely than to consume that food in moderation.

Desserts and Beverages. Fresh fruits, plain gelatin, plain popcorn without the salt or butter, and an occasional small dish of sherbet are in. Other desserts are not. Coffee and tea, with skim milk or lemon if desired, are okay as is an occasional drink of an alcoholic beverage (two to three times per week). The foods in this group to avoid are obvious: cakes, pies, potato chips, ice cream, and that most marvelous invention: the chocolate chip cookie.

Vacation Foods. You need to indulge yourself occasionally. Very well, have any of the following in as great a quantity as you can handle: low-fat boullion, sugar-free carbonated drinks, sugar-free club soda, sugar-free tonic water, coffee, tea, carrots, celery, lemon juice, vinegar, and sugar-free candy. When consuming carrot sticks and celery, *beware* of dips and salad dressings. It may actually be very important for you to indulge yourself occasionally and to do so in an eclectic fashion: The body craves calories, but may also crave certain tastes and certain food groups. More about this in the next chapter.

Rx ——————————————————————————————

Keys to Eating for Cholesterol Reduction

- Remove the skin from poultry.
- Have a fish dish three or four times a week.
- Eliminate eggs from your diet.
- Drink only skim milk.
- Avoid cheese and butter.
- Use tub margarine and polyunsaturated oils.
- Get the advice of a registered dietition.
- Think *lifetime eating plan,* not diet.

Drug Therapy for Lipid Problems

Recent advances in pharmaceutical research are making it even easier to find a pill for a problem. Sometimes drug treatment of lipid abnormalities — elevated cholesterol and/or triglycerides — is necessary. The National Heart, Lung, and Blood Institute stresses the importance of dietary treatment first. Pills can be dangerous. However, if dietary therapy has been followed religiously for six months and the LDL cholesterol (the bad cholesterol) or triglycerides have not substantially dropped, drug therapy will be necessary. We will consider each of the drugs in turn. References are cited in the bibliography. In the following discussion, the brand name is in parentheses.

Bile Acid-Binding Resins. *Cholestyramine* (Questran) and *colestipol* (Colestid) can reduce levels of LDL cholesterol in the bloodstream. They do this by binding themselves to bile acids in the gastrointestinal tract. By so doing, they reduce the total amount of cholesterol in the body, although, remembering our analogy, they do nothing to the number of pickup trucks. The side effects of these drugs are gastrointestinal as well. They produce a lot of stomach gas with belching, bloating, flatulence, heartburn, nausea, and sometimes abdominal pain. They can be constipating. They are not palatable, although a candy bar containing cholestyramine is now available — how American!

Lovastatin. Lovastatin (Mevacor) lowers cholesterol by interrupting the production of cholesterol in the liver. It is more effective in doing so than either cholestyramine or colestipol, and because it is a pill and acts within the liver rather than within the gastro-intestinal tract, it is better tolerated with fewer *apparent* side effects. It *does* have side effects, however. Liver problems are not uncommon and have to be watched for with periodic blood tests. Severe muscle inflammation and kidney problems have also been described with the drug. Use of lovastatin requires frequent follow-up with your physician.

Niacin. Niacin or nicotinic acid, one of the B-complex vitamins, lowers both triglycerides and cholesterol and also increases good cholesterol, HDL cholesterol. Niacin (nicotinic acid) is not to be confused with nicotine. Niacin causes flushing and itching and can cause an upset stomach as well. The trick is to start out with extremely low doses and work up gradually until the proper dose is achieved. Starting out with the proper dose is asking for side effects. Liver tests, blood sugars, and tests for blood uric acid, the chemical that can cause gout, need to be administered if you are using niacin.

Probucol. Probucol (Lorelco) lowers cholesterol, both the bad cholesterol and the good cholesterol as well. Because it reduces HDL cholesterol, because it stays in the body for months after treatment has stopped, and because it may cause some heart abnormalities, I don't use it anymore.

Clofibrate. Clofibrate, marketed as Atromid-S and Abitrate, as well as others, has been used to reduce triglyceride levels. Paradoxically, as it does so, it can increase LDL, or bad cholesterol. It has been used a long time, and with this experience has come the knowledge of increased incidences of diseases of the gastrointestinal tract, including gallstones and cancers. Its use should be very limited. Unfortunately, it is not. It should never be a first line drug to treat triglyceride problems, and it should never be used anyway to treat cholesterol problems alone.

Gemfibrozil.   Gemfibrozil, or Lopid, is used to reduce triglycerides. It also raises HDL cholesterol, a desired result. It is a much safer drug than clofibrate, and the results in reducing the number of heart attacks in large groups of men have been good. It is used to treat triglyceride problems, not cholesterol problems alone. It increases the formation of certain kinds of gallstones, but otherwise, the side effects seem not to be serious.

Fish Oils.   Fish oils which contain **Omega 3 fatty acids** (eicosapentaenoic acid and others) are known to reduce triglycerides and, to a lesser extent, LDL cholesterol. They do not seem to affect HDL cholesterol. Experience with fish oils in capsule form is limited. There may be some evidence in fact that eating fish is preferable to taking fish oil capsules. The real thing is always better than a pill.

To summarize drug therapy of lipid problems: Accepted therapy for high cholesterol includes the drugs lovastatin, cholestyramine, colestipol, and niacin. Of these, lovastatin seems to be the most effective but can have the most serious side effects. Carefully monitored, lovastatin is the drug of choice, if tolerated. Gemfibrozil is the drug of choice for a patient with high triglycerides unresponsive to diet. Clofibrate (Atromid-S and others) should be used only in special situations.

Table 5-3 shows the retail costs of cholesterol-lowering drugs. The usual beginning daily dosage is listed, and the cost in the right hand column is the cost for thirty days' treatment with these usual daily dosages. These costs were obtained from a local pharmacy in Maine and may certainly be higher elsewhere.

TABLE 5–3   Retail Cost of Cholesterol-Lowering Drugs

Drug	Daily Adult Dosage	Cost per Month
Cholestyramine (Questran)	16 grams resin, divided	$76.17
Clofibrate (Atromid-S, Abitrate, and others)	2 g, divided	$27.59
Colestipol (Colestid)	15 g, divided	$54.99
Gemfibrozil (Lopid)	1200 mg, in two doses	$51.39
Lovastatin (Mevacor)	20 mg, single or divided	$47.39
Niacin (generic)	1 g, three times a day	$15.39
Probucol (Lorelco)	500 mg, twice a day	$46.99

HYPOGLYCEMIA One dark night during my internship, an ambulance brought in a man in coma. We examined him closely to find a cause for his coma. He had no evidence of trauma. He had no abnormalities of his pupils. There were no signs of a palsy on one side of the body—nothing to suggest a stroke. There were no signs of meningitis or bleeding into the brain. We drew some blood for tests and then used a standard procedure in similar cases: We gave him a huge dose of sugar by vein. He woke up. His blood sugar test came back exceedingly low. He was not a diabetic taking insulin, yet he had been profoundly hypoglycemic (low in blood sugar). How this happened to him is a fascinating lesson in human biochemistry.

The liver normally stores sugar in energy reserve as packets called glycogen. A normal person has a couple days' worth of glycogen packets to call upon in times of fast. After the glycogen packets are used up, if total starvation or fast continues, the body has to figure out another way to supply the brain with sugar (glucose), the only source of energy the brain can use. The body does this through **gluconeogenesis** (glucose-newly-made). Enzymes in the body convert protein to glucose, the brain is happy, and coma is avoided.

Our patient was an alcoholic. He had a severely diseased, scarred liver, and his cirrhotic liver could only store about twelve hours' worth of glycogen packets. He had been on a binge, had not been eating, and had used up his glycogen. But the enzymes necessary to make new glucose, the factors involved in gluconeogenesis, are exquisitely sensitive to alcohol and inhibited by alcohol. He used up his glycogen reserve and could not make glucose from protein, his blood sugar fell to disastrously low levels, and he lapsed into coma. This is the only case of hypoglycemia I have seen in a nondiabetic patient in the past twenty years.

If hypoglycemia is so uncommon, why do so many people seem to have it? We need to examine the symptoms of an abnormally low blood sugar. All of the symptoms of hypoglycemia, except for one, can be attributed to an excess amount of adrenaline in response to the falling blood sugar. The one symptom that cannot be ascribed to adrenaline is brain dysfunction, and that symptom is caused directly by inadequate energy source, glucose, to allow the brain to function normally. The symptoms attributable to adrenaline are sweating, a sensation of hunger, a feeling of anxiety, a tremor or shakiness to the body, a feeling of light-headedness or a sensation of passing out, and sometimes heart palpitations and a feeling of irritability. These complaints are vague and somewhat common; they can be the results of many conditions, including anxiety and stress, much less "fashionable" diagnoses than is hypoglycemia. Patients presenting with these complaints are sometimes labeled as "hypoglycemic" without further laboratory analysis by the physician. Because the lay press has been so convincing in its assertion that hypoglycemia has reached epidemic proportions, the label is misapplied by friends of the afflicted as well. Why admit to depression, burnout, or midlife crisis when you can be suffering from "hypoglycemia"?

Think of hypoglycemia as a consequence of a

diabetic condition, an alcohol related condition, or a symptom of extremely uncommon diseases.

Low blood sugar can occur *in reaction* to a meal, usually a high carbohydrate meal, and is called **reactive hypoglycemia.** Alternatively, a low blood sugar can occur in the fasting state such as it did with our patient presented above, and that condition is called fasting hypoglycemia.

Let's take the rare condition first: **fasting hypoglycemia.** In addition to patients with severe liver disease and alcohol abuse, rare tumors of the pancreas producing large amounts of insulin can result in very low blood sugar in the fasting state. If insulin produced from within the body can lower the blood sugar to dangerous levels, insulin introduced from outside the body can do so as well. Hypoglycemia of severe proportions is not uncommonly seen in insulin-dependent diabetic patients.

Sometimes after a carbohydrate meal the blood sugar will fall to excessively low levels in response to that meal. This is called reactive hypoglycemia. This kind of hypoglycemia is much more common than fasting hypoglycemia, but is still uncommon. Most often, reactive hypoglycemia is part of the very early set of symptoms of diabetes mellitus. In diabetics, reactive hypoglycemia occurs this way. After a meal high in carbohydrates, the pancreas in patients with early diabetes mellitus responds sluggishly to the large amount of carbohydrates in the meal. Because of the sluggish response just after the meal, blood sugars reach higher levels than normal. Now the body senses these excessively high levels of blood sugar and the pancreas then over-responds. At about three or four hours after the carbohydrate meal, the blood sugar falls to excessively low levels, i.e., *reactive hypoglycemia.*

Reactive hypoglycemia may also be seen in patients who have had stomach surgery, in patients who are following certain fad diets, and in some patients with alcohol-related problems.

Diagnosis of reactive hypoglycemia involves using a prolonged glucose tolerance test. A measured amount of sugar, usually in the form of a sugared cola or "glucola" is given to the patient, and then a series of blood sugars are drawn every half hour to every hour up to six hours after the glucose challenge. The accepted cutoff is usually 50 milligrams per deciliter or lower; however, normal people may reach levels below that without any symptoms.

Treating Hypoglycemia

How should a doctor approach a patient who complains of "hypoglycemia"? If this is a case of running out of steam in the late afternoon, I try to reassure the patient, telling him the information above, and leave it at that. If there is a pattern of reactive hypoglycemia, with the patient-documented symptoms occurring predictably two to four hours after a meal and predictably being more severe after a high carbohydrate meal, I will perform a prolonged glucose tolerance test on the patient. If there has been no stomach surgery, and if the glucose tolerance test is abnormal, I then tell the patient he may have a diabetic condition that merits periodic follow-up. I will as a part of this tentative diagnosis suggest a diabetic diet and weight reduction, if indicated. Hypoglycemia is usually a "nondisease," fraught with subjective signs and symptoms and sometimes with hidden agendas. Diabetes mellitus is not. That is our next topic.

DIABETES MELLITUS

To begin with a story .... I once took care of a patient who raised broiler hens. He was about forty-five years old, lean and fit, and had 20,000 chickens under one roof. He was a busy man. He first noticed something wrong when he began to experience frequent urination at night. This was new for him, as was an increase in his appetite, although he attributed the latter to his vigorous physical work and his "need for energy." He began to carry a gallon plastic container full of cold water around with him while he was doing chores. When he began to crave cold sweetened drinks and consumed colas by the six-pack, his wife began to wonder whether he had "sugar." She called their family doctor who looked in the patient's records and reported to the patient's wife that blood sugar tests done six to twelve months previously had been normal. It couldn't be diabetes.

Weeks later on a particularly hot sunny day, his wife found him unconscious in the broiler barn. The rescue squad brought him to our hospital. The emergency room nurse looked at his dry mouth, parched lips, deep, regular breathing, sunken eyeballs, and made the diagnosis. I got involved when she called me and said:

Come on over quick, Doctor! I've got a guy in diabetic coma.

As obvious as these symptoms of diabetes mellitus can be to health personnel, it is always surprising how inapparent the diagnosis is to patients suffering from its more obvious symptoms. One patient will be diagnosed when recurrent fungal infections of the vagina lead that patient's gynecologist to ask appropriate questions and check a blood sugar. Another patient will be properly referred by an optometrist who finds difficulty in fitting the patient for glasses because of frequent changing of lens prescription. If you follow some simple guidelines, however, you can direct your own health care such that the diagnosis need not be made on the floor of the broiler barn.

Rx _____

Some Facts About Diabetes

- Diabetes runs in families.
- If a family member has diabetes, you are more likely to develop the disease.
- A normal blood sugar twelve months ago does not mean you will never develop diabetes.
- Diabetes is overwhelmingly a disease of middle age.
- Diabetes rarely develops in childhood.
- Although children may have a more serious form of diabetes, 90 percent of diabetes is adult-onset.

- Diabetes can almost always be diagnosed with a simple blood test, long before any symptoms appear.
- Testing the urine for sugar is not a reliable way to screen for diabetes mellitus.
- Reactive hypoglycemia can be an early symptom of diabetes mellitus.
- Most diabetics can be treated with pills.
- Neglecting diabetes can be serious, and fatal.

Diabetes Mellitus—Two Types

There are two categories of diabetics: those who are dependent upon insulin and those who are not. The terms for these two categories are many. Insulin-dependent diabetes mellitus is referred to as **Type I diabetes,** and since this most often develops in childhood, it has been referred to as *juvenile-onset diabetes.* Non-insulin-dependent diabetes mellitus has been referred to as *adult-onset* or *maturity-onset diabetes* and is also referred to as **Type II diabetes mellitus.**

Diabetes Mellitus — Two Types

- Insulin-Dependent Diabetes Mellitus (IDDM), Type I: "Juvenile-Onset"
- Non-Insulin-Dependent Diabetes Mellitus (NIDDM), Type II: "Adult-Onset"

Genetics

The inheritance of both types occurs in a complicated fashion. Type I seems to be caused by some sort of response of the body's own antibody system to a virus infection that inadvertently destroys the insulin-producing cells of the pancreas in the process. The inheritance of type I diabetes seems to be an inheritance of the susceptibility for this antibody destruction, rather than an inheritance of the disease itself. Whereas certain forms of muscular dystrophy will be inherited in a predictable fashion in families with the abnormal gene, those families carrying the gene for susceptibility to type I diabetes cannot be so easily advised about mode of inheritance. At least two factors are necessary to develop type I diabetes: the gene for susceptibility to disease, and exposure to the virus or viruses responsible for the inappropriate antibody destruction of the pancreas.

Likewise, inheritance of type II diabetes depends upon many factors, and its inheritance cannot be easily predicted. In addition to whatever genetic abnormality there might be, environmental factors play a great role in the development of type II diabetes; most notably, obesity and our American diet. A simple statement says it best: Diabetes mellitus runs in families in an unpredictable fashion. Continued surveillance for diabetes mellitus in such families is wise.

Before we leave the topic of genetics in diabetes mellitus, I want to make an important point about an unusual complex of diseases: **polyendocrine glandular failure.** About 15 percent of patients with type I diabetes will get an inappropriate antibody destruction to other glandular tissue, such as the thyroid gland, the adrenal glands, the cells in the stomach that help to absorb vitamin B-12, and certain muscle tissue. Some of these patients having problems with many endocrine glands in addition to the pancreas will show inheritance of these problems with family genetics analysis. The message is a simple one: If you have diabetes mellitus, especially type I diabetes mellitus, be on the alert for the development of problems with other endocrine glands.

A short story to illustrate .... One of the nurses at the hospital told me rather dejectedly that her internist had diagnosed her as having an underactive thyroid, pernicious anemia, as well as the diabetes mellitus she had been contending with for some years. I took care of her mother, a known diabetic. I called her mother in the next day, ordered screening tests for other endocrine dysfunction, and diagnosed hypothyroidism (an underactive thyroid) and Addison's disease (failure of the adrenal glands) in the mother.

What Happens in Diabetes Mellitus

The tissues need glucose for energy. **Glucose,** a form of sugar, is the energy that runs the factories of the cells. All tissue, except the brain, can use other energy sources, such as the fatty acids that are stored in that spare tire you're trying to get rid of. The brain cannot; glucose is the only energy source the brain can use. Insulin, produced in certain cells of the pancreas, called *islet cells* or *beta cells,* is crucial to glucose use by the body's tissues. Insulin allows glucose to get inside the cells where it can be used, and insulin also allows the body to store excess glucose for use later on — that is, to store it in the form of glycogen in the liver, as we mentioned before when talking about our alcoholic patient and to store it in the form of fat in adipose tissue. Depending upon whether some or all of the beta cells wither and scar or are destroyed by antibodies that should be attacking a virus, a patient may have mild or severe diabetes mellitus. Lack of sufficient insulin causes profound elevations in blood sugars, resulting in a marked increase in urination, thirst, and weight loss from loss of fat tissue and muscle and from loss of body water. Eventually, with no glucose available to think on, the brain functions improperly and coma ensues.

To summarize: Lack of sufficient insulin causes profoundly high blood sugars but no sugar (glucose) available for the brain to function. Coma is the result. But coma results also from *too much* insulin. Excessive amounts of insulin produce very low blood sugars. In this condition also, there is no glucose for the brain and coma results.

Symptoms and Diagnosis

The three cardinal signs of diabetes mellitus all doctors are taught are the three "polys": polyuria, polydypsia, and polyphagia — that is, abundant urine, abundant thirst, and abundant appetite. Frequent infections — especially skin infections and fungal infections between the folds of the skin, under the breasts, or in the vagina — may hint that the disease is present. In children, bedwetting, apathy, fatigue, and weight loss may hint that diabetes is the problem. Because of problems prescribing glasses or because of recurrent problems with gum and teeth infections, the optometrist or the dentist may make the diagnosis.

The laboratory standards for diagnosing diabetes mellitus are quite simple: A normal blood sugar in the fasting state is less than 115 mg/dl. A diabetic has a fasting blood sugar greater than 140 mg/dl on more than one occasion. Sometimes diabetics may have normal fasting blood sugars and will need to be tested with a glucose meal. A blood sugar between 140 and 200 two hours after a carbohydrate meal is strongly suspicious of early diabetes mellitus; a blood sugar of 200 mg/dl or more two hours after a glucose meal is diagnostic of diabetes mellitus. It is important to remember, however, that *there is no single level above or below which a patient is declared diabetic or normal.* The determination of some abnormal blood sugars in an individual dictates close surveillance for the development of the disease. For example, a 28-year-old man with two fasting blood sugars of 140 should not have checkups only every five years as discussed in Chapter Four. This patient should have blood sugars checked about every six months.

Treatment of Diabetes Mellitus

The single most important facet of treatment of diabetes mellitus is not insulin: Anyone can write a prescription for insulin and syringes. The most important aspect of treating a diabetic is *patient education.* Doctors do not have time and, in most cases, do not have the knowledge necessary to educate a diabetic. Those patients with insulin-dependent diabetes mellitus (type I) should receive extensive education sufficient to manage their own disease except in times of acute medical emergency requiring hospitalization. Put simply: *Diabetics should be in charge of managing their own disease.* Several diabetic clinics throughout the country do an excellent job of such patient education: for example, the Joslin Diabetes Center in Boston, the International Diabetes Center in Minneapolis, the Diabetes Clinic of Grady Memorial Hospital in Atlanta (along with many local

American Diabetes Association affiliates throughout the United States).

Patients with non-insulin-dependent diabetes mellitus (type II) do not necessarily need to go to such clinics, but do require extensive diabetic teaching to learn about the importance of diet, how activity affects diabetes, how to recognize when a diabetic condition is worsening, how to recognize low blood sugar, and the proper approach to foot care. Foot care is important because the poor circulation associated with severe diabetes can cause marked deterioration of the tissues in the feet.

Diet

As mentioned above, most patients with type II diabetes are obese. Weight reduction is *mandatory*. For these people weight reduction is much more important than any carefully measured diabetic diet. In fact, achieving ideal body weight, followed by an adherence to a reasonable diabetic diet, will be all the therapy necessary to treat a diabetic condition in many cases. Diabetic diets are not simple, and when compounded by the need for weight reduction and the extreme importance in diabetics of cholesterol restriction, such diets can be quite complicated. They require the expertise of a dietitian or registered nutritionist. To obtain the services of a registered dietitian, simply ask for them. Say to your doctor, "I want to see a registered dietitian."

Those patients using insulin therapy — patients with type I disease — face an additional complicating problem in their diets: the need for special timing of eating. Meals have to be spaced and must include afternoon and bedtime snacks so that the distribution of the daily calories over the course of the day is constant and regular. Only in this way is an adequate dose of insulin arrived at.

Some other points about diet: Diet exchange lists are available from both the American Diabetes Association and the American Dietetic Association and usually from most hospital dietitians. There is never any need to buy special, expensive diet foods or "diabetic foods." Finally, a common misconception insulin-dependent diabetics have about diet: Commonly patients who develop a mild illness and are not eating properly will stop insulin therapy in the mistaken belief that if they are not eating, they do not need insulin. The dose may need to be reduced, but the insulin should never be stopped. Physician's advice is mandatory in such situations.

Drug Therapy For Diabetes Mellitus

Treatment of diabetes mellitus with agents to lower blood sugar is a topic somewhat controversial. I will tell you what I do.

Patients with type I disease necessarily will be on insulin. If they are not acutely ill, I will have our nurse-practitioner teach the patient and a family member how to draw up and administer insulin, and I will then get the visiting nurses to supervise this in the home for as long as is necessary. Such patients will be directed to the hospital dietitian and to the hospital's patient education programs dealing with diabetes mellitus and its management. If the type I diabetic has especially "brittle" diabetes — that is, diabetes featured by wide fluctuations in blood sugar and very difficult to control blood sugars — I will suggest, even insist, that such a diabetic go to a teaching center such as the Joslin Diabetes Center in Boston. These patients will then learn all about their disease: how worsening diabetes is manifested, how to manipulate their insulin dosages depending upon their own blood sugar testing at home, how to manage their diet depending upon intercurrent minor illnesses, and how to care for their skin and feet.

Common Home Blood Glucose Testing Kits

Glucometer II, Blood Glucose Monitoring System with Memory	$195.00
Glucometer M, Blood Glucose Meter	$200.00
ExacTech Meter Package	$225.00
Accu-Chek II, Blood Glucose Monitoring System	$135.00
Lifescan One Touch	$220.00
Glucoscan 3000	$170.00

TABLE 5–4   Pills Used to Control Diabetes Mellitus

| Generic Name | Brand Name | Average Daily Dose | Retail Cost per Month | |
			Generic	Brand
Tolbutamide	Orinase	1 gm	$5.69	$11.99
Chlorpropamide	Diabinese	500 mg	$7.39	$27.39
Acetohexamide	Dymelor	500 mg	$8.99	$13.39
Tolazamide	Tolinase	500 mg	$14.99	$20.39
Glipizide	Glucatrol	10 mg	N/A	$10.69
Glyburide	Diabeta Micronase	5 mg	N/A	$10.39

Type II patients, typically obese middle-aged patients, who are symptomatic — that is, present to me any of the above symptoms we have talked about — are initially treated with insulin and with a weight reducing, calorie restricted, *carbohydrate restricted* diet. In those cases of real miracle, when the patient actually adheres to the diet, gets down to an ideal body weight, and strictly follows diabetic diet guidelines, insulin therapy can be stopped, and no further drug therapy will be necessary. If weight control cannot be achieved, I will keep the patient on insulin unless he or she refuses to take insulin, in which case I am forced to use one of the drugs in Table 5-4.

For patients who have no symptoms but whose diabetes is diagnosed by abnormal blood testing, here too diet therapy may be enough. If it is not I will use one of the oral preparations in Table 5-4.

Elderly patients with mild diabetes mellitus present a special problem. They often eat poorly and at irregular times with varying caloric intake. I treat them gently, do not use insulin, and tend to use a very short-acting drug such as tolbutamide rather than one of the longer-acting drugs such as glyburide or chlorpropamide.

Complications of Diabetes Mellitus

A detailed discussion of the many complications of diabetes is beyond the scope of this book. A few points however do deserve emphasis.

Insulin and the oral preparations do lower blood sugar. Excessive amounts of the drug, especially in combination with fasting, or starvation, can lead to exceedingly low blood sugars (hypoglycemia) and coma. That is why our high school first baseman, a juvenile diabetic, always carried a candy bar and would never share it.

Diabetics have a markedly increased tendency to develop cholesterol deposits in the blood vessels. Diabetics frequently will have heart attacks at a much earlier age than normal individuals, and they are much more prone to developing stroke. Problems with arteries in the limbs, especially the leg arteries, are especially common in diabetics. But early treatment helps. Good control of diabetes can often help the diabetic avoid many of these complications.

Not only does diabetes cause damage to the large blood vessels, therby leading to stroke, heart attack, and poor circulation in the extremities, but also diabetes attacks the tiny blood vessels, the microcirculation. These small blood vessels — which help the kidneys to function, feed the nerves of the body, and nourish the retinas — can, when diseased, lead to disastrous consequences. Nerve problems in diabetics can lead to painful extremities, leg cramps, impotence, and problems of bowel motility. Kidney problems are a late complication, but a problem that must be watched for and anticipated. It is especially important in diabetics to treat promptly — indeed to avoid altogether — urinary tract infections. Remember, these are all problems that can be anticipated and, in many cases, be avoided given proper therapy. Treatment of diabetes mellitus is one of the best examples in medicine of how early, effective, and lifelong treatment can matter to the patient.

Eye Complications in Diabetics

Diabetics frequently develop complications involving the eye. Cataracts, glaucoma, retinal bleeding, and partial or complete loss of vision are much more common in diabetics. These complications occur regardless of whether the diabetic is on insulin therapy or not. It is mandatory that every diabetic get periodic examination by an ophthalmologist. An optometrist's examination is not sufficient. (An *ophthalmologist* is a medical doctor who specializes in diseases of the eye.) One of the greatest recent breakthroughs in diabetic therapy, since Banting and Best discovered insulin in 1921, is the development of laser treatment of diabetic retinal problems. Spot-welding of leaking blood vessels in the retinas of diabetics has spared countless diabetics partial or complete loss of vision.

In summary, the diabetic patient should remember three important points:

1. Diabetes is a disease best managed by the patient, not the doctor.
2. A wealth of educational resources for the diabetic patient exists, usually free of charge.
3. Routine visits to the ophthalmologist are mandatory for the diabetic, regardless of whether one has eye symptoms or not.

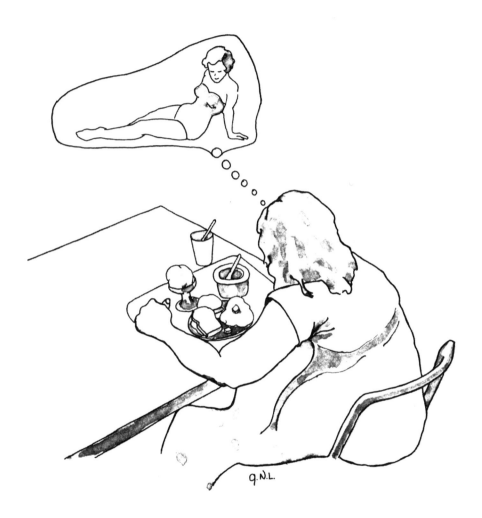

6

Fat Man's Misery

One of the most exciting climbs in the Northeast is Maine's Tumbledown Mountain. The climb does not require any technical skill, the ascent is fairly brief, and the work involved is minimal for the spectacular view afforded at the top. The view at the summit from open ledge includes a pristine lake near the summit, and all of that wonderful Maine out there. The climb in some parts is nearly vertical as one ascends a series of ledges. At about midway in the ascent, the route travels through a narrow crevice steeply pitched and provided with old iron rungs. The climber, surrounded on four sides by rock, pulls himself up through fifteen feet of narrow crevice. The crevice is called "fat man's misery."

And how miserable it *is* to be fat. You do not conform to the American dream. You are a living, breathing, quivering target for the moral judgments of others. You are judged self-indulgent, gluttonous, and lacking in self-control.

To wake up one morning finding yourself thin —that is one American dream. We wish to be *made* thin, passively stripped of fat without ever having to refuse one chocolate chip cookie. (Indeed, now liposuction seems to offer us that chance, for a fee). Advertising appeals to this shared fantasy every day of our lives, telling us of new, effortless, quick, miraculous schemes to shed weight. Having lost our will to work for a goal, to sacrifice for some long-range gain, we search for the pill, the painless approach, the miracle. We are suckered into total immersion language courses, where we can become filled with nouns and verbs in a week, finally realizing fluency in French. We forego the soap operas on television to watch the classics (abridged, of course) so that we might painlessly earn the title of intellectual. In school we sacrifice basic disciplines for "relevant" courses and get paid off with easy credits for social protest, glib rhetoric, and intensive self-absorption. We go around once in life, grabbing all the gusto we can. *Self-denial is anti-American.*

As a society we are doing better. There are more joggers today than there were twenty years ago. There are certainly more dieters today than there were a hundred years ago. But, in the main, as a society we are still not doing very well. The rest of the world continues to view us as "fat Americans", over-indulgent, all-consuming.

DEALING WITH OBESITY

When is one considered obese or overweight? Table 6-1 can serve as a rough guide. It does not apply to the weight lifter or the football player but for the rest of us, it will do. Quite simply, if you are over the upper limit for your height, you are *overweight*. If you are overweight by more than twenty percent of your ideal weight, you are *obese*. If you weigh two times your ideal weight or more, you are *morbidly obese* — morbid in the medical sense of carrying with it serious health consequences.

When our sedentary, consuming American way of life renders us disgustingly plump, we steel ourselves for a few weeks of crash dieting. First, buy the glossy books. Then drink gallons of water, taking joy in urinating away all that fat. A little "Diet revolution," then "fat-free forever," now to "carbo-cal," and then some "immune power" please. We wash some windows, take the stairs instead of the elevator, split a few sticks of wood, and imagine the pounds rolling off. After a few weeks of such torture and praiseworthy demonstration, telling all of our friends that "this is it", we find that we have not lost an ounce. We may have even gained a few pounds. The brow furrows knowingly, the eyes squint against the blinding insight: Wisdom whispers to us, "it's hormonal." Hat in hand, we load our flesh into the car, and go off to the doctor.

"It's hormonal. Tell me the secret of losing weight. Make me thin," we say. "No it isn't. And there are no secrets. I can't make you thin," is Honesty's answer.

We have an incredible capacity for self-delusion. Our self-image is couched in pleasant euphemisms: We are stocky, plump, heavy, big-boned. We imagine ourselves filled as much with potential as we are with fat. With a secret smugness we imagine how much more sexy, or youthful, or athletic, or efficient, we would be if we *wanted* to shed that twenty pounds.

TABLE 6–1   Height–Weight Chart

Height (in shoes)	Small Frame (lbs.)	Medium Frame (lbs.)	Large Frame (lbs.)
		Men	
5 ft. 2 in.	112-120	118-129	126-141
5 ft. 3 in.	115-123	121-133	129-144
5 ft. 4 in.	118-126	124-136	132-148
5 ft. 5 in.	121-129	127-139	135-152
5 ft. 6 in.	124-133	130-143	138-156
5 ft. 7 in.	128-137	134-147	142-161
5 ft. 8 in.	132-141	138-152	147-166
5 ft. 9 in.	136-145	142-156	151-170
5 ft. 10 in.	140-150	146-160	155-174
5 ft. 11 in.	144-154	150-165	159-179
6 ft.	148-158	154-170	164-184
6 ft. 1 in.	152-162	158-175	168-189
6 ft. 2 in.	156-167	162-180	173-194
6 ft. 3 in.	160-171	167-185	178-199
6 ft. 4 in.	164-175	172-190	182-204
		Women	
4 ft. 10 in.	92-98	96-107	104-119
4 ft. 11 in.	94-101	98-110	106-122
5 ft.	96-104	101-113	109-125
5 ft. 1 in.	99-107	104-116	112-128
5 ft. 2 in.	102-110	107-119	115-131
5 ft. 3 in.	105-113	110-122	118-134
5 ft. 4 in.	108-116	113-126	121-138
5 ft. 5 in.	111-119	116-130	125-142
5 ft. 6 in.	114-123	120-135	129-146
5 ft. 7 in.	118-127	124-139	133-150
5 ft. 8 in.	122-131	128-143	137-154
5 ft. 9 in.	126-135	132-147	141-158
5 ft. 10 in.	130-140	136-151	145-163
5 ft. 11 in.	134-144	140-155	149-168
6 ft.	138-148	144-159	153-173

But losing weight is hard work, and requires total honesty. It seems all but impossible. Very few achieve weight control. Why? This whole business requires choices, tradeoffs, personal responsibility, and the here-and-now as opposed to some nebulous concept of the future and longevity. Weight control involves changing behavior. *That* is always difficult. Another reason for the seeming impossibility of dieting is that it *does* require honesty. And the diet doctors are not being honest with you. **It is almost impossible to lose weight and keep it off through dieting alone.**

Too often gimmicks, tricks, deceptions, and lies appeal to us. Hard work never does. Too often we exist only to be gratified. As Americans, we have an over-abundance of processed junk foods which deliver more calories per bite than anything un-American. This, together with our American sedentary way of life, compounds the problem. We are hardly a nation of walkers or bike riders; we are not even a nation of joggers. There are roughly two hundred million Americans of voting age. Only one-tenth, or 20 million Americans, get regular exercise.

There is some evidence that obesity in infancy predisposes a person to intractable obesity in adulthood. One is fat both by virtue of the number of fat cells in the body (and the consequent capacity to store fat), and the amount of fat stored in each cell. In other words, a person with few fat cells has little capacity to store fat. Overfed infants are endowed with more fat cells for life than normal infants. Those who have been obese since infancy may be partly correct when they say that "everything I eat turns to fat." If they eat more calories than they expend, the excess calories may more easily be stored as fat. Here are some symptoms of our preoccupation with food:

- a baby is not deemed healthy unless fat
- relatives are often offended if second helpings are refused
- family get-togethers focus around food and calories
- to be fat is to be prosperous
- to be skinny is to be unhealthy, and "off your feed"

Fat people behave differently than those of normal weight. Fat people are much less active. Video recordings of children in playgrounds have carefully shown this to be true. Fat people have different feeding controls than normals. They have no compensatory period of abstinence after overeating as normals do. They tend to eat on time cues from the clock rather than when they are hungry. They eat fewer meals per day, bunching calories into one or two large meals, a practice known to enhance fat storage in the body. Finally, the obese have a self-defeating set of rationalizations which most of us share to some extent: Food is used as a tranquilizer, as a reward, to assuage anger and injustice, or to please others.

The rationalizations are incredible, and silly, if we examine them honestly. We believe that if we eat while standing, eat hurriedly, eat alone, on the sly, or don't really enjoy it while we eat, then it can't be fattening. If we load up before the big event, we are sure we'll burn it off. We consume artificial sweeteners as though they themselves will melt away the fat. We skip breakfast and later overcompensate. We prepare for an anticipated missed meal by gorging ourselves beforehand and then, incredibly, manage not to miss the meal after all. We eat for two.

We eat food in tidbits until we have consumed far more than we normally would because we believe that the whole is not the sum of all of its parts. And when in the end we eat more than we burn up in calories, we get fat, and we look around for someone else to blame. This seems to be true, whether we have been obese for life or have awakened at forty wondering what has happened.

The Social and Health Consequences of Obesity

Obese people are discriminated against. They lose out in relationships, in sex, in job applications, and in medical care (through inadequate examinations obstructed by layers of fat and through complications from surgery). They lose out in life. Obesity is a health hazard. Like the arthritic, the obese person is easy prey to quacks and gimmicks. There is a solution, but it is not easy, seldom written about in diet books, and expensive in cost of effort. To get to the solution, we need first to understand how we think about obesity, how we get fat, and why diets don't work. Yes, you're impatient. You want the solution — *the gimmick*. The solution is in Chapter Seven. But we have to get there first. Bear with me.

As animals, we have many primitive notions so instinctive that they lie far beneath consciousness. Consider the matter of territory, for example. So basic is our sense of ownership of property that our hackles are raised when a car turns into our driveway, even before that intrusion reaches our consciousness. Pride in ownership runs far deeper than any sense of accomplishment. We are filled with instinct — the pregnant woman's nesting behavior, the mother's protectiveness, the urge to plant in the spring and hoard in the fall —and much of this instinctive behavior still serves us well. One such notion does not.

The idea that obesity brings health and strength, once serving us well, now only does us harm. We still believe, falsely, that the fatter the baby the healthier, the more robust the pregnant mother, the better things will be. Weight loss is sensed, in some primitive place in our minds, as a threat to health, and to strength. Matriarchs must be fat as a condition of office. Fat will protect us against disease and famine. In harder times it did; when we hunted for supper, those who could store a few extra meals ahead were better off.

Today, obesity is neither fashionable nor healthy. Where once famine and malnutrition weeded out the thin, obesity with its attendant chronic diseases of diabetes, high blood pressure, heart disease, and stroke now kills off the fat. With a skeletal system designed for 120 pounds now burdened with 30 pounds more, is it any wonder that obese people complain of fatigue? And what is the burden on the heart? Blood pressures rise, cholesterol is deposited more liberally in the blood vessel system, and the heart runs down. The middle-aged obese person is a prime target for heart attack and stands a very poor chance of surviving one. Among other problems, should he suffer a cardiac arrest his massively obese chest will insulate the heart against any effective external cardiac massage.

A twenty to thirty percent increase in weight above normal doubles the risk for heart disease, triples the risk for gallbladder problems, and makes the possibility of developing type II diabetes many times more likely. Arthritis of the weightbearing joints is much more common. Obesity is a special hazard in pregnancy since high blood pressure and toxemia are more prevalent in obese women.

An adequate physical examination is almost impossible to perform on obese patients. The heart sounds are distant and muffled, as are the breath sounds, and the abdominal and pelvic organs are distanced by layers of fat and impossible to palpate. Anesthesia is more dangerous in obese persons. Layers of fat several inches deep hamper surgery.

The psychological damage from obesity is just as profound. Many obese people are depressed. They may suffer from loss of esteem, harbor self-doubt and feelings of inferiority, and live in the fantasy world of "if only's." Obese people may have a significant amount of self-hate, ranging from disgust to self-destruction. In extreme cases, feelings of isolation lead to more over-eating, more obesity, and a slow suicide.

Becoming Obese

How do we become obese? Unfailingly, it is a matter of time and arithmetic. Over the years, consuming more calories than we burn, those excess calories are stored as fat at 3500 calories per pound. To maintain an ideal body weight, we need to consume in calories roughly fifteen times that ideal weight in pounds. For a moderately active mother weighing 120 pounds, this amounts to 1800 calories per day. How can she, with every intention to the contrary, become obese ten years hence?

Consider this hypothetical case. Once a week, over and above her careful 1800 calories per day, she indulges herself. She has a Big Mac one week (557 calories) and a hot fudge sundae the next week (580 calories). Add a couple of doughnuts (500 calories), half of a small pizza (900 calories), a large dipped Dairy Queen cone (450 calories) . . . and so it goes. Her weekly indulgence becomes a part of her life. At each tally of 3500 calories, a pound of flesh is stored away. At this rate, she gains a pound every six weeks, or eight and a half pounds a year. In ten years she weighs 205 pounds. *It happens all the time.*

Now, she quietly rages inside. She wants it off overnight and is terribly frustrated at her fat's tenacious clinging.

What might she have done differently? We will talk more about this later, but had she walked for an hour three times per week, with everything else constant, she would have burned an additional 750 calories per week and would have had room to spare for her weekly indulgence. Or she might have dieted one day a week at 1200 calories for that day, giving herself the margin of her weekly indulgence in another way.

Finding Your Own Equation

Fortunate people seem to do this adjusting and compensating by instinct. I had a dear friend, a restaurateur, who weighed 125 pounds all of his life. Well, almost all of his life. A diminutive Frenchman, he was filled with energy, darting about his restaurant like a humming-bird. First to the Caesar salad, then to the pâté, now he is pouring wine, then he is listening to a complaint, now he's greeting guests at the door. This Frenchman consumed whatever he wanted without an afterthought. He loved his Bordeaux, never refused the Camembert, and specialized in desserts. His customers were not so fortunate.

The rest of us must, it seems, replace instinct with hard work. This learning of in-come and out-go must be learned privately, by personal experience, for each human machine is different, using and storing fuel in different ways. No one formula can work well for everyone. That is why, after all, crash programs and gimmicks usually fail. The weight is gained back because there's no learning taking place. One is too busy, hoping for miracles.

The learning is difficult. We gorge ourselves,

quickly step on the scales, and find we haven't gained an ounce. We remain smug in our secret victory until three days later, when our weight shoots up, seemingly out of control. It's not fair, we scream inside, having forgotten the indulgence of three days before.

We grow tired of watching, counting, and denying, as geese might tire of migrating if they were only given the option. We find no time for exercise. Life is exercise enough. We relax the guard. The weight creeps up again.

Is there really a solution? Yes there is, but not in gimmicks, not in tricks, not in fad diets, *and certainly not in drugs.* But let's look first at some of the treatment failures.

Drug Therapy for Obesity

Pills have no place in the treatment of obesity. In fact, *treating obesity with drugs is dangerous business,* although physicians prescribe them all the time. **Amphetamines,** taken lifelong, probably do lower the set point (the brain's thermostat for weight), increase the body's metabolic rate, and curb appetite. They are fiercely addicting, dramatically raise blood pressure, and are associated with marked increases in the rates of stroke and heart disease. **Diuretics,** drugs to induce urination, rid the body of salt water and, since a pint is a pound, cause you to lose pounds of fluid. But not an ounce of fat is lost. As soon as the drug is stopped, the body avidly holds on to salt and water, the fluid reaccumulates, and the weight is regained.

Various preparations of **thyroid hormone** are prescribed by diet doctors (also known as quacks). Thyroid hormone speeds up the metabolism and causes a breakdown mostly of muscle rather than of fat, leading to moderate weight loss. When the drug is stopped, the weight is regained, and usually more weight is regained than was lost through the use of the pill. **Digitalis** preparations, used to treat various forms of heart disease can, as a side effect, cause a loss of appetite, usually when a patient has accumulated too much of the drug in the body. This toxic side effect, the loss of appetite, is still used as an appetite suppressant. This is *very* dangerous business. Toxic amounts of digitalis cause abnormal heart rhythms, often leading to cardiac arrest.

Injections of a hormone obtained from human placenta, human chorionic gonadotropin, may produce (through a placebo effect) weight loss if combined with severe calorie restriction. Human chorionic gonadotropin was the basis of the **Simeons Diet.** When two groups of patients were compared, both on the same calorie-restricted diet with one group getting placebo injections and the other getting injections of human chorionic gonadotropin, the two groups lost equal amounts of weight.

The best advice is to avoid diet drugs and doctors who prescribe them. Every community has its doctor who, because of his failure to keep up, because he has allowed his knowledge to become dated, relegates himself to the fringes of medicine. Among these doctors on the fringe are the diet doctors who readily prescribe diuretics, amphetamines, digitalis, and thyroid hormone to desperate people who will go to any extreme to lose weight. The patients always go secretly. And because the patients *know* that this is a quack brand of medicine and that they are participating in it, they rarely inform on these doctors. Nor do they ever sue them. Diet doctors are gradually being replaced by big business, an improvement only in the sense that the fad diets presently marketed are far less dangerous than the drugs pushed by the diet doctors.

Fad Diets

Fad diets are designed for one purpose: to sell diet books and therefore make a lot of money for the author. If any one of the fad diets really worked, that diet would put the others out of business. Fad diets contain some bizarre gimmick together with restriction of salt, sugar, carbohydrates, or all three, to produce a profound diuresis (increased urination) and the appearance of quick weight loss. Because weight loss through a conventional diet is frustratingly slow and because calorie counting is boring, the fad diets do the counting for you. To say it another way, they do the thinking for you. I have trouble with that approach. Those diets which *are* well balanced nutritionally and *can* be followed indefinitely include the Weight Watchers Diet, the Diet Work Shop Diet, Redbook's Wise Woman's Diet, Dr. Glenn's Once and For All Diet, and the Nutri-System Diet Plan. Some other fad diets can endanger your health. *A few are life-threatening.*

But, if you are obese, you need a diet you can live with forever. More importantly, you need to learn how to think for yourself. Bouncing from one gimmick to another, from carbohydrates to fats, from Atkins to Glenn to Simeons, teaches you nothing. And most importantly *you need to learn the value of exercise.*

Diets restricting the amount of carbohydrates, or diets which promote a high protein intake, have problems of their own. These diets are designed to produce **ketosis,** a chemical change in the blood suppressing appetite, possibly dangerous to those with a diabetic condition or with gout. These diets also pay no attention to fat intake; cholesterol and saturated fats are consumed in excess quantities. And because they restrict certain food groups, they are unsound over the long term. A well-balanced diet, moderately restricted in calories and designed to take off about a pound per week, is much preferred. But it is not the entire answer. That comes later. We will get to it.

Self-Help Groups

The most successful of all self-help groups, Alcoholics Anonymous, has shown the way for many obese people. Realizing that obesity, like alcoholism, is an illness, groups such as TOPS, Weight Watchers, Overeaters Anonymous, and Diet Work Shop can be quite successful when combined with proper diet and exercise. One finds support, understanding, and shared insight. The support these groups can offer an obese person is substantial. No one understands a problem like one who has experienced it. The level of sophistication varies from group to group but better to swallow pride than pastry. Join up. I have found only one problem with self-help groups.

A few years ago, when I served as a physician

advisor to one such self-help group, I noticed a curious thing. Members programmed themselves for failure so that they could stay in the group. What was happening was this. Obese members, all women, would energetically lose a profound amount of weight over the months they belonged to the self-help group. Meeting weekly, they would weigh in, demonstrate their self-control, and earn lavish praise. When they approached their goal, and the time when they would no longer need the group, some of them began gaining weight. They admitted that they had been lonely, isolated, and the group had given them their only real sense of community, the one social outlet in their lives. *Threatened with the loss of that community, they remained fat to belong.*

Behavior Modification

Changing one's approach to food is excellent advice as an adjunct to dieting. The idea is to follow a list of rules (which *you* make up), rules designed to keep one's mind focused on the job at hand. I read about a great lesson in behavior modification. An obese woman decided that she would simply wash every bit of food she ate. She would eat whatever she wanted but she would wash it first. The effect was wonderful! The chocolate cake crumbled in the wash water. The tuna sub became soggy and inedible.

There are less drastic ways of modifying your behavior. You can keep a list of everything consumed each day and tally up the calories. You can eliminate favorite foods from your house. You can keep in the house only foods which need to be prepared before eating. And, following Richard Watson's advice, you can never eat processed foods. You never skip breakfast. Never eat alone. Weigh in every morning. Never eat standing up, or in the kitchen, or while watching television. When feeling angry, frustrated, or depressed, substitute an activity or strenuous exercise for eating. Never clean your plate. Forget about the starving hordes. *And what starts out as a rule will end up as routine.*

Fasting

During my tour of duty in the Army, there was a time when our small hospital faced a crisis. We didn't have any inpatients. The colonel called us doctors in and lined us up against the wall. "Either you guys increase the census, or Washington's going to close this place," he warned.

We had our orders. We looked for any and every patient we could admit. A few days later, a woman weighing 390 pounds came into my office. "If I could just get my weight down," she said, "I know I could keep it off."

I admitted her to the hospital. As an Army dependent, she was entitled to free medical care. I began her on a total fast, except for 300 calories per day of egg whites designed to spare her from protein (muscle) loss. She received minerals and vitamins daily. I visited her twice a day, as did the Army dietitian, and we measured her serum electrolytes and liver function on a weekly basis. We followed her blood pressure and heart rhythm four times a day. We ran periodic checks on her urine to be sure she wasn't cheating on us.

After three days of this, she was no longer hungry. In five days, she was euphoric. On weekends, she was allowed home for a couple of hours of visiting with her family. Her family supported her, heaped praise upon her, and encouraged her in her struggle. The weeks rolled by.

In seventy days she weighed under 300 pounds for the first time in ten years. She was ecstatic. She hadn't cheated; she had done it; fasted, lived on egg whites and pills, and made it! Could she stay another month, she begged? Of course! She could stay two months if she wished. It would keep the colonel happy.

After four months in the hospital she had lost 140 pounds. At the day of her discharge, we had a little party for her on the ward (diet cola, celery stalks, carrots, things like that). She cried, thanked everyone, hugged me and all the nurses, and took her diet plan home to her family.

I never saw her again as a patient. She never even made her first follow-up appointment a week later.

Months later, I saw her at a distance in the commissary. She had gained all of her weight back. She wouldn't look at me.

We could have kept her hospitalized for another six months. We could have maintained her on a 1200 calorie, well-balanced diet in the hospital and the Army would have paid for it. We could have kept her away from her family for a year at the Army's expense, having her prepare her own meals in the hospital under the supervision of a dietitian. And maybe, just maybe, she would have beaten her illness in the end. *But how practical is that?*

Liquid Protein-Sparing Diets

These diets are a variation on the theme of fasting. The idea is that you put a powder in the blender and mix water or skim milk and drink it three times a day and you get enough protein to prevent you from breaking down muscle. You get calories restricted enough so that you lose weight. You get a supply of vitamins, minerals, and electrolytes so that you avoid the problem of heart arrhythmias that the early liquid diets presented. (The Cambridge Diet, one of these early liquid diets, had such problems and is dangerous.) Newer programs, Optifast, Medifast, and Health Management Resources (HMR) are now in vogue. They are very expensive. A six month program of Optifast costs about $2,800. The pharmaceutical company marketing the powder will release the powder only under a doctor's continued supervision. Patients enroll in the program, report to a hospital clinic weekly, and, while on the liquid diet, learn about proper diets to be followed down the road. They learn about exercise and are followed weekly by dietitians, psychologists, and physicians.

As the patient reaches his or her ideal weight, the diet is changed from the liquid protein-sparing formula to a well-balanced calorie-restricted diet. However, the patient continues to go to the clinic. That is a good idea. Some learning needs to take place.

The programs are very expensive. Sometimes third party payers will pick up about fifty percent of the cost — *sometimes.* I have a close friend who has lost seventy pounds in such a program. I am betting that he will make it for one reason only. They have taught him the value of exercise. For most, however, the program is limited in access, prohibitively expensive, and not reasonable. To use a quote from W. Somerset Maugham in another context: "It is easy to be a holy man on the top of a mountain."

Surgery for Obesity

Surgery for the morbidly obese is fraught with complications. Stomach stapling and gastric balloons are designed to reduce the size of the stomach so that the patient fills up quickly and enjoys satiety for the first time in years. In some cases, the balloon leaves the stomach and blocks the intestines, and emergency surgery is necessary to relieve the obstruction. There are case reports of patients with gastric bypass, gastric stapling, or with jaws wired shut, sipping heavy cream through a straw, never losing an ounce. Surgery on a 300 pound patient is risky. There can be a three to four percent mortality. Two percent of these surgery patients will get stomach ulcers, another seventeen percent will need a second operation to make a smaller pouch. A significant number of these patients become profoundly depressed when the tranquilizing effect of large food intake is lost. When a 30-year-old mother of two died two days after gastric bypass surgery in a small hospital near us, that hospital stopped doing any further such surgery.

A REASONABLE APPROACH

We need to take a break for a moment. It's easy to get high blown, overly authoritarian, in this business. We would do well to remember something Robert Pirsig said, "The trouble is that essays always have to sound like God talking for eternity, and that isn't the way it ever is. People should see that it's never anything other than just one person talking from one place in time and space and circumstance. It's never been anything else, ever, but you can't get that across in an essay."

In other words, what follows is advice from one doctor. You need to incorporate it into your own approach — *do your own thinking* — make your own adaptations. Remember the patient with the peanut butter? Remember the patient who wanted me to keep him alive on *his* terms? That's the idea.

Maintaining your ideal body weight demands a drastic change in daily routine and lifestyle. A sensible diet, a change in behavior, help from others, and most importantly daily exercise are essential to any weight loss/maintenance program. You need to reflect on how such a change will affect family, friendships, job, and leisure time. In other words, one needs to reset priorities. An effective program will cost about an hour a day. Will you allow your daily routine to permit it? From whom will you take the time? Who and what will you sacrifice?

The effort to lose weight may take a year or more, and to maintain ideal body weight will require effort for the rest of your life. It will mean saying "no" to dessert and deeply wounding your hostess. It will mean being antisocial at parties when the other chubby hands reach out for drinks and dip and you do not. It will mean feeling and looking ridiculous when you exercise and all your fat goes up when you are coming down. It will mean saying "yes" to yourself and feeling guilty, and saying "no" to yourself and feeling pain. It will mean the realization that there are people, even those who love you dearly, who would like to keep you fat forever. In their eyes, being fat means being weak, and being weak means permitting yourself to be controlled by others. And even those who love you dearly are often reluctant to give up that control. Losing weight is *never* painless.

You will need to decide that obesity is a disease, that you are different from normal people who are thin, and that you cannot eat what they eat and expect to look like them. It may mean pretending that you are a diabetic or a heart patient and must be on a special diet because you have a "health condition." You will need to conduct yourself differently to stay alive. You will need also to convince yourself that you haven't the vaguest notion of how you look and that your *feelings* will never tell you how much you weigh, how much weight you have lost, or how you appear to others. You will need to decide that hunger itself never burned up a single calorie, that you have a terrible self image, and are at the same time both too harsh with yourself and too lenient. You will need to rely on *objective* data: the scales, clothing sizes, the mirror, pictures of yourself. It will mean not trusting yourself with your own assessments until you have won the battle objectively.

The first step in this approach is to get a good physical examination to quiet that part of you still doubting, that part that still believes your problem is a glandular one, some bizarre metabolic disease which no doctor has yet diagnosed. While getting the examination, get medical clearance for vigorous exercise and get a target weight from your doctor. Don't rely on your own judgment of what weight feels best. Begin to mean business.

Imagine for a moment you are living in a foreign land. You are working at a modest job, earning a modest living, living among the people, doing whatever it is they do. There are no fast food chains, few processed foods, and prices for beef are astronomical. Wonderfully, by common agreement, television is turned off across the land every Thursday night. Your modest income does not permit dining out, does not allow beef, butter, or even a dozen eggs a week. You walk everywhere. You bike to work. You begin to measure your happiness by sunsets rather than by steaks. You have cereal for breakfast, homemade soup for lunch, and bread, cheese, and garden vegetables for dinner. Three times a week you have meat, and it is always either chicken or fish. At first you miss hamburgers, pizzas, and the evening's anchorman telling you how to interpret the news. Soon, however, you conform to this drastic change in lifestyles. *There is no alternative.*

The Keys to Control

After the doctor's visit, get a well-balanced diet of about 1500 calories for men and about 1200 calories for women, a diet designed to shed one to two pounds per week *maximum*. Forget about vitamins and your concerns of malnutrition. Get the diet from your doctor or from a registered dietitian and make sure you understand it. Eliminate all processed foods from your household. If the rest of the family wants cookies, let them go out for a treat. Have no desserts in your house — none. Never skip breakfast. Never skip any meal. Never snack. Never cheat, no matter whose party it is or whose feelings are going to be hurt. Remember, you have a disease, a "health condition." If you need help and company, join a self-help group or form one of your own. Or weigh in at your doctor's office at least once a month.

Change your behavior immediately. Weigh yourself everyday no matter how painful. Do it in the morning. Get out pictures of yourself in a bathing suit at top weight. Look at them frequently. Keep a list of everything you eat for a week and total up the calories. Dispel the notion that eating certain foods will *cause* weight loss. Even if you *don't* like cottage cheese, it still has calories. Learn the difference between appetite and hunger. Learn to say no to appetite demands. Learn that hunger won't kill you. Pause when you find yourself at the brink of failure. Inevitably, you will find yourself there at that brink, staring at the doughnuts and wondering, do I or don't I? At the brink, usually something bad happens. Clouds cover reason. Resolve is postponed until after the doughnut. A full stomach and guilt prevail.

You *must* stop at the brink everytime, step back from it, and consider your priorities. Look at where you are, how petty and foolish this battle really is, although it appears overwhelming from the inside. Then decide what to do.

Finally, convince yourself that daily exercise is central to any weight loss program. When you need convincing, turn to Chapter Seven and read it again. And that gets to our secret of weight loss — my "gimmick." If you believe nothing else in this book, believe that *you cannot diet successfully, lose weight, and maintain your ideal weight without a regular sensible daily exercise program.*

For Heaven's sake, be gentle with yourself. Be

satisfied with the best you can do. We come in all shapes and sizes and, within limits, cannot improve upon Nature. Nor should we want to. What a boring place this world would be if we were all as thin as Mia Farrow.

And now we've reached the end of this chapter, and it is time for exercise. It seems appropriate here to close with a quote from Richard Watson:

"Fat represents the nagging triviality, the utter banality, and the inevitability of ordinary reality that separate us from what we think we want to be. Render out some of that fat. Get down to the muscle. Bare yourself to the rising wind . . . it really does not matter much to the rest of us what you do, so long as you don't hurt anyone. But if you don't do something you will be proud of later on, it will matter to you."

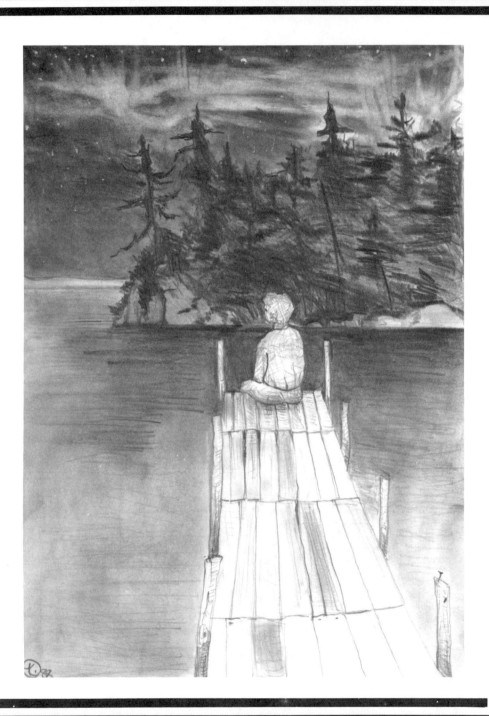

7

The First Prescription: Exercise

"Man is an animal, and his happiness depends on his physiology more than he likes to think. Unhappy businessmen, I am convinced, would increase their happiness more by walking six miles everyday than by any conceivable change of philosophy."
Bertrand Russell

Two weeks of late summer fly-fishing in Quebec — that
had been the whole idea. He had found a small outfitter
in Baie Comeau who had taken him by float plane to a
remote lake in northern Quebec — a lake with one camp
only, his camp, for the two weeks with no one, nothing,
to intrude upon the hundreds of acres of forest surrounding him. What he did not know was that after
dropping him off at the lake, his pilot, on the return
flight, had died in a crash. No record of his guest's
whereabouts remained.

The man's days of escape and relaxation quickly
passed. But now the float plane was four days overdue.
The man paced along the dock, stamping his feet
against the morning frost, repeatedly scanning the
skies for his outfitter's float plane. He thought of the
meetings he was already missing, the contracts to be
signed, the customers to win, the business to conduct,
the money to be made. He swore softly. He could no
longer be interested in fly-fishing. The rise-form of the
trout had no fascination for him. He needed to get back.
He was overdue.

And now, at twelve days overdue, he began to
panic. He had not seen one single plane overhead. The
September wind hinted at winter. The snow geese
began heading south without him. The man was soft,
civilized, entitled to comfort, to accommodation. He was
out of his element, without defense. He had no control of
time.

Against the wind's chill, against his panic, he
went into the camp and started a fire in the woodstove.
He had to get hold of himself. He had to take stock of
what he had. The camp came fitted with an ax, a
hatchet, and a small bucksaw. With the abundance of
blow-downs, mostly pine and spruce, but dry nevertheless, he would not want for firewood. He would not
freeze to death. He had the woodstove, the camp's
cooking utensils, and plenty of knives. He had matches
and old newspapers, plenty of bedding, warm clothing,
and good boots. He had his fishing equipment, which
could serve him until the lake froze. But he hadn't a

firearm. He could not hunt, and with winter hardening on the lake, he would do no fishing either.

But he had no food. He had run out of food, just. He searched the cupboards and every nook and cranny of the camp and found only a box of stale rice and an old jar of peanut butter left there by a prior fishing party. He didn't like peanut butter — he especially didn't like old peanut butter, somebody else's peanut butter. He put the jar and the stale rice aside.

He was not a reader. He had brought no books with him. But in the spare bedroom he found two old volumes. One, quite substantial, yellow, and dog-eared, its cover partly torn away, held the complete works of W. H. Auden. The other book, more slender but equally old, was entitled Uses of Plants by the Chippewa Indians by Frances Densmore. The book had no pictures and as a guidebook, was, he thought, utterly useless.

He banked the fire, blew out the kerosene lamp, and crawled into his sleeping bag, tired and hungry. He would fish all the next day, he thought, dry the fish, and stock up for winter. He would survive.

He fished the next day until his arm ached, pounding the water until the sun went down and the fish would no longer rise to his fly. It was that time of year when the trout are busy with another call and he managed to net only fourteen fish, each a pound or so. These he gutted and split and hung on a makeshift rack to dry. He saved the two largest trout for his supper.

The next morning, he found the drying rack in shambles and his fish gone. Furious at the animal that had made a fool of him, he tried to channel his anger into the business of cutting firewood. He stacked the wood under the cabin, sat on a stump in the morning sun, and collected his corporate senses.

With new resolve he packed the hatchet, the boots, and the Densmore book and paddled the five mile length of the lake to the headwaters and feeder streams. He beached the canoe, lay on his belly in the grass next to the sandy stream flowing into the lake, and watched the brook trout finning slowly upstream, intent upon instinct. Away from the banks of the stream, he cut armloads of alder saplings. Then he made a fish-weir upstream with the saplings, a trap narrow upstream at its top and wide downstream at the base. With one sapling he fashioned a spear. He circled to the downstream end of the brook and then threw rocks ahead of him upstream to frighten the fish into his weir. Enervated by their spawning, the brook trout milled in the weir until he could spear them. He filled the bottom of his canoe with the speckled trout. Then, excited by his small victory, he climbed the rise of the land carrying the Densmore book. At the top of the rise, eight miles from camp, he found what appeared to be, from the description in the book, a swaying stand of Sedum purpureum — "live forever". He checked Densmore, following excitedly with his finger, and then dug with his hands into the mossy earth and found the crisp white tubers. He filled the front of his shirt with them.

He forgot about meetings. He forgot about business deals and clients and making money. He thought about living and about how to live and about what was important to him after all. He watched the migrating geese and studied them from the woods as they fed in the mudflats. He watched how they took off, how they needed to spread their wings and run a length to launch themselves into the wind. He constructed a long goose-trench, a ditch shallow enough that the geese would go in after bait with the security of peering over the top, ever on guard, a trench narrow enough to prevent the geese from spreading their wings and launching before he could catch them. He baited the trench with some of the rice, caught and killed several of the geese, and smoked them together with the fish in the woodshed he had converted into a sturdy mammal-proof smokehouse.

To the west, a brisk twelve mile walk from camp, he found wild caraway and hoarded their parsnip-like roots. And on another such hike he was greeted with an entire field of Daucus carota — Queen Anne's lace — and with his hatchet in his hands he dug for hours their white, carrot-like roots. He stored his precious parsnips and carrots in boxes of sand in the cold bedroom. From the rafters of the camp he hung mint and elderberry and labrador tea.

He played with making a simple peg snare and, when he thought he had it perfected, he made several at some distance from the camp and baited them with the rice and with the old, stale peanut butter. He smoked the spruce grouse he caught in this way and, with the squirrels he snared, he made jerky and a crude pemmican using the meat, the fat next to the skin, and some dried berries he had gathered.

He began to walk for the sheer joy of it. The acres of forest surrounding his camp became as familiar to him as his house in the city. He played with calling back and forth across the lake to the barred owl. He became aware of his body, the stretch of his limbs, the power in his hips, the lift of his shoulders. He became aware of his own self-sufficiency.

Bundled against the north wind, sitting at the end of the dock watching the grand display of northern lights, he wondered to himself if he wished that no one would ever rescue him. He had discovered Auden, who had saved his sanity. He had his companion in Densmore, who had saved his very life. And he had himself.

"Laurence, you look terrible!" they exclaimed when they got him back to civilization. "You're skin and bones! You need a bath. And a shave. And a decent meal."

And so he was back. He was back to civilization, back to that place where the walking of three blocks on a city street feels like a marathon, where a meal consists of grease and dough, where beauty is defined by the frame of a television screen.

Would he hold on to his new-found simplicity, this healthy discipline that was no longer imposed upon him? Would he seize and keep this drastic change in lifestyle he had learned to love? Could he continue to maintain his new priorities? Will you have him fat again? Will you have him lounging on the couch, numbly watching television, hardly thinking for himself, hardly living? Would you have him forget Auden? Will you have him think of Densmore as a silly memory? And what about you? How would you have yourself live?

He is stranded in the north woods and *must* exercise, you say, must use his body, simply to survive. Discipline imposed from without is not part of the real world, you say. But do *you* want to survive? For how long? How well? *Exercise is the key to surviving, and surviving well.* That's what this chapter is about.

Consider a list of risk factors for heart disease, conditions which make it more likely that you will suffer a heart attack:

Hypertension	Cholesterol abnormalities
Obesity	Cigarette smoking
Inactivity	Dietary habits
Stress	Family history
Diabetes	

Of these, all except heredity can be improved upon or eliminated by a vigorous exercise program.

IS EXERCISE GOOD FOR YOU?

Heart disease aside, is exercise really beneficial? Does it do anything other than sell customers expensive running shoes and fancy jogging gear? And what about the arthritis of the hips that runners can get, and what about the people found dead by the side of the road, and what about all of that car exhaust, and what about, what about? We will look at the medical complications of vigorous exercise later on, but first let's talk about how exercise and good health are linked and why exercise is so essential to dieting and weight reduction.

Diet and Exercise

We doctors used to have a very simplistic idea about the problem of obesity and dieting: Take in more calories than you need and you get fat; take in less calories and you lose the same amount of fat; fat people who say they don't eat much are lying. Simply take in the right number of calories and you will get to your desired weight — that was the idea.

The entire obesity-exercise problem is much more complex. One workable theory to explain part of these complexities is the "set point theory." There is some good research evidence that the brain has a kind of thermostat setting for body weight — a setting to keep the individual at a particular weight which we call the set point weight. This **set point** is probably determined by inheritance, early feeding in childhood, the kinds of foods we eat now, and, most important to our present discussion, by physical activity. The set point obviously varies. It explains why, in part, two individuals differing by fifty pounds in weight can eat exactly the same diet and each maintain his or her weight. Or more simply, people may be naturally heavier or lighter depending upon the set point. The body employs several tricks to maintain the set point weight. One of these is physical activity. Observe children in a playground, and you will find that obese children are less active than their thinner classmates. The heavier children move with economy.

Appetite, or lack of it, is another trick the body uses to maintain the set point weight. And, finally, the rate at which the body burns stored fat and sugars, the rate of metabolism, is turned up or turned down by the body's mechanisms to maintain the set point. We have inherited this from our caveman ancestors. Here is the essence of the theory: During times of feast, when there are plenty of trout for the catching and the fields sway with caraway and Queen Anne's lace, the savage stuffs himself completely, stores the excess calories, decreases his appetite, and increases his metabolic rate and activity in an effort to maintain his set point weight. What he cannot eat in food he buries in the sand or smokes in his woodshed. When the woodshed and the sandbox are empty and his food is nearly gone, when winter is hard upon him, his body attempts a hibernating mode, trying to conserve what few calories are left to him. His metabolic rate slows down, his appetite increases, and hunger rages from within him. His body tenaciously holds on to the set point weight however it can.

And so it is with the well-intentioned dieter. The dieter also goes into a hibernation-mode. He or she feels the effects of a lowered metabolic rate: its extreme lethargy, its raging appetite, and the frustrations of little or no weight loss.

How To Adjust the Set Point

We know of only a few factors affecting the set point. Dietary sugar and fatty foods tend to raise the set point. It is so important to avoid simple sugars and fats in the diet, not just because of their caloric load, but because of their adverse effect on the set point. You can lower the set point by strenuous physical activity or by cigarette smoking. People who combine vigorous exercise with dieting are successful for that reason. And that is why ex-smokers experience weight gain.

Exercise is much more important to a diet than for its burning of calories. That is the message. *Exercise strongly influences the lowering of the set point.* The type of exercise is as important as its duration. Aerobic exercise is the only kind of exercise that can lower the set point. We will talk in a moment about kinds of aerobic exercise and about the degree and duration of exercise desired, and examine a sensible exercise program a bit later. But first let's consider a benefit of exercise other than the maintaining of an ideal body weight.

Exercise and Longevity

Almost every group, from Harvard graduates to Masai tribesmen, has been studied for the effects of exercise on health. Each of these studies strongly suggests that habitual exercise reduces the risk of heart attacks. Just as importantly, the studies show that a sedentary "couch-potato" existence is also a major risk factor for developing heart disease. Exercise protects against diet-induced hardening of the arteries. It elevates the good (or HDL) cholesterol and lowers the bad (or LDL) cholesterol levels and, in laboratory animals, exercise markedly reduces cholesterol deposits in the major arteries of the body.

One of the most important studies in this regard, the study of Harvard alumni by Paffenbarger over ten years ago, showed that sedentary men were at a sixty-four percent higher risk for heart attack than their classmates who exercised in the amount of at least 2,000 calories per week. This study showed that not only did exercise reduce the risk of heart attacks but also promoted longevity. As physical activity increased from 500 calories per week to 3500 calories per week, death rates continued to decline steadily. And a similar study in Finnish men showed that active middle-aged men lived two years longer on the average than sedentary middle-aged men.

Cynics counter with images of that extra two years in a nursing home. But the bargain is far more than this. It has to do with living your allotted threescore and ten to enjoy your accomplishments, your family, and your grandchildren rather than leaving all of this at age fifty because of a massive heart attack. And still more: It has to do with becoming aware of yourself and of your body, and of what your body can do, of feeling the power in your hips, the lift of your shoulders, and of feeling self-sufficient, of being able to take care of yourself as though you were lost in the woods. The fisherman stranded at the lake will not live forever. But he can take care of himself. *He is in charge.*

I will tell you a story about a patient. . . . This patient, age forty-two, came to me because of chest pain with exertion. Testing proved that he had severe coronary artery disease, critical deposits of cholesterol within his coronary arteries obstructing the flow of blood there. Studies also showed that this was an inoperable condition — there was nothing the surgeons could do for him. He was young and in the prime of his life. He was accustomed to being active, accustomed to skiing and swimming with his teenage daughter and son. He despaired. He felt as though his life were already over. What could he possibly do?

There was plenty to do, I told him. He was twenty pounds overweight. He could start a cholesterol-lowering diet, an American Heart Association phase II diet, and discard the burger-fries-potato chip habit. He could take medication to control his angina, and a medication to help drive down his cholesterol. He could begin some carefully monitored, supervised exercise with limits as defined by a treadmill stress-test.

He took the pills, he followed the diet, and he sacrificed the fast-foods. Most importantly, he began an exercise program and stuck to it religiously. In a supervised way, he exercised while watching his Boston Red Sox struggle for the pennant.

A year and a half later, his cholesterol has fallen from 276 to 159 mg%. He no longer experiences angina despite decreasing the amount of medication. His tolerance for exercise has markedly improved. He can now exercise forty-five minutes a day at a very high workload without any distress. He has lost the twenty pounds, feels as though his life is just beginning, *and he always wears a smile.*

Before You Exercise!

The medical complications of exercise belong to two groups, those that are orthopedic and those that are not. The orthopedic problems — muscle strains, ligament tears, stress fractures — can usually be avoided through prudence and common sense. We will consider those orthopedic problems later.

The nonorthopedic complications of exercise can be more serious. The story which begins Chapter Five, for example, illustrates a chief danger of exercise, sudden death through undiagnosed coronary heart disease. Exercise increases the workload on the heart. A heart diseased by cholesterol may not get sufficient blood supply during this increased work. Abnormal heart rhythms and even permanent damage to heart muscle can result. Strenuous exercise, even during a simple viral illness, can cause problems. Jogging while suffering with the flu, for example, can promote a viral infection of the heart muscle with sometimes serious consequences.

Exercise can provoke an asthmatic attack in people who are prone to asthma. This kind of "exercise-induced asthma" is not uncommon. The use of drugs to control this type of asthma in world class athletes has caused considerable controversy during the Olympic Games. It has complicated the drug testing procedure and analysis.

Sometimes a type of allergic reaction may complicate strenuous exercise. With this complication, the athlete develops a generalized, hives-like skin rash with the intense itching and burning of the skin sometimes associated with asthma. I remember a fabulously talented young hockey player whose promising career was ended by a severe form of such an exercise-induced skin allergy (cholinergic urticaria).

Abnormalities in menstruation are very common with vigorous regular exercise, probably because of a loss of total body fat. These menstrual irregularities resolve with a decrease in training and with weight gain. No complications of reproduction function have been described. Some women who cease menstruating while continuing serious training may be in danger of a thinning of the bone matrix such as occurs after menopause, so-called **osteoporosis.** It is well to have a physician caring for you, a physician who treats athletes, is trained in bone physiology, and can keep watch on possible problems of bone density and demineralization of bone.

Strenuous warm weather exercise brings with it the danger of **heat exhaustion** and **heat stroke.** Heat stroke is an extremely dangerous problem, signaled by the cessation of sweating and the abrupt onset of mental confusion, profound weakness, and collapse. We all remember the 1984 Summer Olympics in Los Angeles and the finish of the women's marathon. Such overheating can be avoided by drinking large amounts of water before and during exercise in hot weather and by avoiding extremes of temperature, exercising, for example, early in the morning or at dusk.

Exercise in winter weather carries with it the danger of **frostbite** and **hypothermia** (a decrease in body temperature). Runners, cross-country skiers, winter climbers, and snowshoers may all be subject to cold injury. Because it is so common, let us consider frostbite more closely.

Frostbite usually appears in the extremities: the ears, the fingers, the toes, the nose. The patient experiences a stinging, quickly followed by numbness. The frostbitten area looks white and pallid. One should only treat frostbite by gentle rewarming with *warm* water, not hot water and certainly *not* with the application of ice. Frostbite can be serious: Every doctor in training remembers cases of alcoholics found asleep on a park bench during cold weather, with frostbitten toes requiring amputation.

A case of frostbite cost a hockey team a very important game and, at the same time, made me a very unpopular team physician. With the score tied at two, our team's star mentioned that he couldn't feel his toes. This game was played in the old days, you see, when hockey was played outdoors with the north wind tearing across the blue lines and with a crowd of only a few parents in arctic coats, parents who were frostbitten themselves. The coach called me into the locker room. I had the boy take off his skates. Eight of his toes looked white and lifeless, like something found in Madamme Tussaud's. I took the boy out of the game, the team lost its best player, and the enemy from across town scored two quick goals and left happily. I left as quietly as I could.

Orthopedic Problems of Exercise

Everyone worries about whether weight-bearing types of exercise such as jogging or running will eventually result in a wear and tear kind of damage to the joints, a damage we call **osteoarthritis** — the wear and tear arthritis we are all subject to after the age of fifty. There are no final answers about this. I will give you mine. It is better to limp at seventy from arthritis than to die at fifty from heart disease.

But I do suggest prudence in this matter. Marathon-running is not only senseless but foolhardy for someone who weighs 190 pounds. That person is asking for trouble. Yet someone who weighs 190 pounds and more prudently runs thirty miles a week will rarely be seriously injured.

The most common kinds of orthopedic injuries, musculoskeletal injuries, occur because of overuse. Common sense is best — a careful warming up period and a graduated exercise program involving small increments in exercise — is well advised. You cannot undo in a weekend what it has taken you forty years to become. Keep in mind:

- If it hurts, stop.
- Life is long.
- Injuries heal.

Stretching and sensible warm-ups will avoid many injuries. And when injuries do occur, a modest decrease in intensity, and alternate forms of exercise, can often treat the problem successfully.

A Checkup For an Athlete

I recommend an exercise program wherein you will burn at least 2,000 calories a week in an aerobic fashion. And I recommend before you begin this program that you have a medical clearance.

If you are young and apparently healthy you should have a good physical examination from a physician who will take a good history as well. You need a physician who looks for risk factors such as family history of heart disease, high blood pressure, stroke, and sudden death. You should have the routine screening blood tests we talked about earlier including a cholesterol/lipid profile, blood sugar, and blood count. If the history is not suggestive of increased risk and your physical examination is normal and the routine testing is fine, then you are free to begin. And if this testing is not all normal, it is all to your good to have found out.

A story . . . . I was confronted with a scowling eighteen-year-old son whose parents (he thought) were overly protective. They insisted he get this checkup before committing himself to a mountain climbing expedition. It appeared he was already in excellent physical condition. He had connections, knew someone who knew someone, and had landed a position with the Sherpas in Nepal to help pack supplies to a base camp for an assault on Everest. He was ready to go at once, and who at eighteen isn't? His parents had insisted just on this one checkup.

The picture of health, he sat on the examining table in his shorts looking like an ad for Fruit-of-the-Loom. I admit to the temptation: Why not rubber stamp the whole thing and get him out of the office?

He had one hell of a heart murmur. I was amazed that no one had ever heard it before, surprised that no one had ever mentioned it to the patient or his family. The patient said that he couldn't remember anyone ever listening to his chest before. The murmur came from an abnormal enlargement of heart muscle, a kind of abnormality that can result in sudden death in young athletes. He had a very abnormal electrocardiogram. A sonar image of his heart, an **echocardiogram,** demonstrated the abnormally enlarged, bulging, obstructing heart muscle which had produced the murmur and which might, with strenuous exercise, lead to sudden death. With proper medication, and after strenuous exercise testing proved that he could make the trip, he got to Nepal and to the base camp at Everest.

If You Are Over Thirty-Five . . .

Older patients should have the screening checkup mentioned above and should *definitely* have some sort of exercise stress-test. Any patient of mine over thirty-five years of age, regardless of risk factors or lack thereof, will have an exercise stress-test before beginning any regular exercise program.

In an exercise test the supervising physician takes electrocardiograms while the patient is exercising on some sort of machine, most commonly a moving treadmill. The exercise-work is graded according to the speed of the treadmill and the work can be increased by increasing both the speed and the inclination. We are always surprised at what this kind of exercise stress-test might reveal. Let me give you an example . . . .

Death of a Salesman . . . Almost

Our group of internists performs its stress tests at our local hospital. After ten years of doing so, the hospital needed a new **electrocardiogram monitor** — the machine that records the electrical wave impulses from the patient's heart during the exercise test. Our old machine was worn. Buying a new machine like this is never simple. One does not go down to the nearest mall and pick out a machine. You have to suffer through the sales pitches. None of the salesmen, of course, will simply give you a price and sell you a machine. They want to show you the product. They have to go through their routine and then they make "a deal" with you and you get into one of those horrible bartering situations that most of us hate. The salesman wheels in his machine, he attaches it to his own chest and he jumps up and down. He shows you what a beautiful picture of heart wave recordings you can get even though he's bouncing up and down. He smiles and raises his eyebrows at you and gives you fawning looks and makes you think that if you don't buy the machine from him it will be the equivalent of selling your little sister to the Libyans.

One such salesman came by with his machine. His was the best, he said, the most fantastic machine of all, he said, and we wouldn't believe the wave forms we would see on the oscilloscope and so on and so on. He took off his shirt and the technician shaved the spots on his chest where the electrodes were supposed to go. She pasted the electrodes on and then attached the electrodes to the machine. I turned on the treadmill and he stepped on the moving belt and started walking at a very slow pace, all the time giving his pitch as he was walking, smiling at me and making me think that he was my best friend. And, with only *mild* exercise, his electro-cardiogram abruptly became terribly abnormal. The technician gasped, I flipped off the treadmill motor, and everyone became very quiet and very serious. The salesman himself was thirty-five years old and had never had a checkup. He had been experiencing a type of pressure in his chest when he exercised, a pressure he had called "gas", and had never given it a second thought. Until that moment, that demonstration to us of his new machine, he had been a prime candidate for sudden death.

If you're over thirty-five, get a stress-test before beginning an exercise program. *It's always worth it.*

And after the testing and the medical clearance, you can make the decision to get to work and take charge of your life. Now you can get up from the grass, turn away from the stream, and set your eyes on the ridge up over and begin the climb. And when you reach the top of the ridge you will find wild caraway and Queen Anne's lace and much more. You will find yourself. *It will amaze you.*

ABOUT AEROBIC EXERCISE

Aerobic exercise, the exercising of large muscle groups repetitively for long periods with an increase of the heart rate to roughly eighty percent of its maximum level, is the *only* kind of exercise I prescribe. Read Cooper's books as cited in the bibliography. Convince yourself.

In considering aerobic exercise we have four parameters in question: the intensity of aerobic exercise, its frequency, its duration, and the type of aerobic exercise.

Intensity. Intensity of exercise is measured by the heart rate one achieves during aerobic exercise. Intensity is not measured by how fast you run a mile, how quickly you swim a lap, or how steep the hill is you climb. Intensity, for our purposes, is measured only by heart rate. Chart 7-1 enables you to determine the effective training range, heart rate, and intensity, for your age. Best conditioning occurs at a heart rate of seventy to eighty-five percent of your maximum heart rate. Maximum heart rate is approximately 220 minus your age; one simply takes seventy to eighty-five percent of that to get a training range. The chart eliminates the arithmetic. For example, at age forty-five, your training range would be 125 to 150 beats per minute. At age sixty, the training range would be approximately 112 to 137 beats per minute. As you become conditioned, you will need to work harder at whatever it is you are doing to achieve a heart rate in the effective training range. When you first begin exercise, you will need only to climb a flight of stairs to get your heart rate up to about 130. As you become fit, you will need to do more work to raise your heart rate to this level. In the ensuing months, as you

CHART 7–1   Effective Training Range By Age

Best fitness occurs with an intensity of exercise that brings the pulse rate to approximately 75% of the maximum possible heart rate. The fastest your heart can beat is approximately 220 beats minus your age. The graph below eliminates the arithmetic. For example, at age 50 the most effective training range is between about 120 beats per minute and 145 beats per minute.

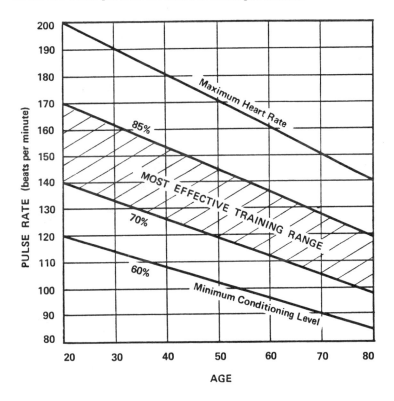

exercise and become more fit, you will need to do a good bit more work to stress yourself. *That is the whole idea.*

There are two ways to take your heartbeat during exercise: the cheap method and the expensive method. Figure 7-1 demonstrates the cheap method. The model has her fingers on her carotid pulse. Feel for your pulse yourself; you will find it easy to locate. Count the beats in fifteen seconds, multiply by four, and you have your pulse rate for a minute. This can become difficult to do

FIGURE 7–1   Touch Method for Checking Carotid Pulse

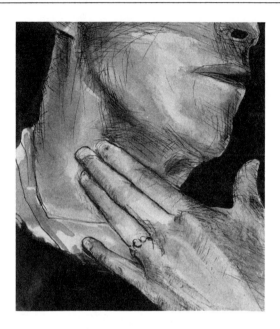

during exercise, but it can be done with practice. Eventually, you will get a sense, just from the feel of your body, whether you are stressing yourself adequately or goldbricking.

Expensive methods of pulse taking are for sale. NordicTrack (address in the bibliography) sells some very good pulse monitors and distributes a Finnish model which is especially reliable.

Frequency.   If *intensity* is the first consideration of exercise, *frequency* is the second parameter to consider. A *frequency* of exercising seven days a week is ideal — but there are children to cart here and there, and Little League games, and teachers' conferences, and the in-laws always dropping in. To achieve cardiovascular fitness, a frequency of four days a week is minimum.

To summarize thus far: You are going to begin an exercise program you will commit yourself to at least four days a week, and ideally seven days a week.

During that exercise program you will work toward an intensity of exercise sufficient to raise your heart rate to the training range we talked about. For these two variables, intensity and frequency, the kind of exercise and the duration of exercise are not important.

Duration of Exercise. How long should an exercise period be? Now things get a little more complicated. Your goal is to *eventually* work up to an expenditure of 2,000 calories per week. Chart 7-2 shows various kinds of aerobic exercises together with a very approximate estimate of calories used per hour for that exercise. Looking at that chart, you can see that when you eventually become conditioned, and are thus fit to spend 2,000 calories per week, when you reach that

CHART 7–2 Calories Burned/Hour of Exercise

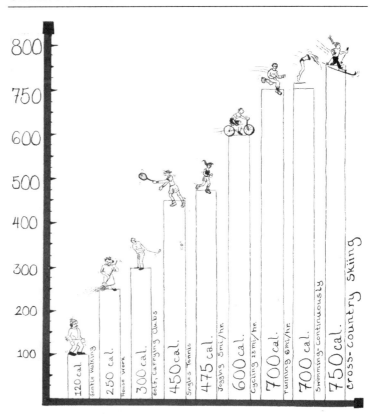

point, *what* you do will dictate *how long* you do it. You can play five hours of singles tennis per week or you can cross-country ski for two hours and forty minutes per week; both activities will expend the same amount of energy.

Example:

   2,000 calories per week desired
Tennis, singles: 5 hours
   400 calories per hour used

   2,000 calories per week desired
Cross-country skiing: 2-2/3 hours
   750 calories per hour expended

Anyone who tells you that swimming, running, or cross-country skiing are the best physical conditioners possible is giving you a qualified statement without giving you the qualifications. They are the best conditioning exercises *for the time expended.* If you want to walk four miles an hour for one hour every day, God bless you. I have elderly patients who do just that — in fact, every night, on my way home from the hospital, I see two of them, husband and wife, holding hands, out for their evening walk. They have been doing it together for years, seem always young and fresh and excited, and are committed to surviving for each other.

Certain occupations are strenuous enough without adding a program of jogging. It would be folly to suggest to a farmer or woodsman that he buy a bicycle. But the rest of us overestimate the amount of real work we do on the job, no matter how physically exerting it seems to be for us. Few jobs will raise heart rates into the training range consistently for twenty minutes or longer. Similarly, doubles tennis, golf, bowling, and baseball, although excellent recreational exercises, are not sufficient for the job we have in mind. There are always exceptions. I have a patient in his seventies who plays eighteen holes of golf everyday, seven days a week, always at a brisk walk, always carrying his own clubs, and sometimes adding another round of nine holes to his routine of eighteen. He is fit, healthy, and fine. He is the *exception*.

Types of Aerobic Exercise.   If you are fortunate enough to have the leisure time, I suggest walking. Walking at an intensity sufficient to raise your heart rate into the training range is the best of all kinds of exercise: It is simple, easily accessible, requires a minimum amount of equipment, and is always fun, regardless of the weather. A Colin Fletcher type of walking is best of all (see bibliography).

If you suffer from the constraints of time, shorter periods of higher intensity conditioning are imperative. Jogging and running, while simple and accessible, are jarring and pounding types of activity, tough on diseased joints and low backs, and rather more damaging to the muscles and skeleton. Cycling and swimming are nonweightbearing activities which are best for those with joint diseases. However, they are subject to weather and inconvenience. Cross-country skiing is recommended by most to be the best kind of aerobic exercise. But it too has its shortcomings; it is very difficult to ski in West Texas.

Don't get caught up too much in *what* you do. My most successful patients vary the type of exercise by season, by impulse, or by changes in the weather. But they do *something*. They are active. They enjoy that activity. It is fun. As Richard Watson recommends, be concerned first with the *form* of your life and decide upon *content* only after that. Or consider Colin Fletcher:

> *First, make sure the ways and the means remain just that. They will always be threatening to take over.*

My most successful patients cycle, weather permitting, cross-country ski when the snow is just perfect, and jog in between. It is *exercise* that has become a part of their lives rather than the entering into a log book the number of miles run this week.

To summarize, you need to expend at least 2,000

calories per week in some kind of aerobic exercise as outlined on Chart 7-2. The intensity of that exercise must be sufficient to raise your heart rate into the training range as determined by Chart 7-1. The frequency should be at least four times per week and preferably everyday, and the duration must be long enough to expend 2,000 calories per week.

Swimming Example:

Intensity — heart rate in the training range.

Frequency — five times per week.

Duration — 35 minutes per session.

$$\frac{2,000 \text{ cal./week (need to expend)}}{5 \text{ days/week}} = 400 \text{ cal./day}$$

$$\frac{400 \text{ cal./day}}{700 \text{ cal./hour (swimming)}} = .57 \text{ hours}$$

.57 hours $\times$ 60 minutes = 34 minutes/day (swimming)

You don't need to get this complicated, nor have you to relearn algebra and deal in fractions. The point is this: If you haven't the leisure time for a brisk long walk everyday you need a high intensity type of aerobic exercise for a shorter period of time, everyday, to achieve the results we are talking about. To diet, to lose weight, to control your diabetes or your high blood pressure, to minimize your risk of heart disease, and to live longer, and more importantly, to live more fully, *you must develop an exercise program that works for you.*

Exercise Machines

What if you can't jog because of your arthritis? What if you hate running? What if your low back condition prevents you from cycling? And suppose the nearest swimming pool is twenty miles away, with public swimming only from 5:00 a.m. to 7:00 a.m. You want to exercise. What to do? You may need to buy a machine. What kind of exercise machine is best?

The best sort of exercise machine requires aerobic exercise, is low in cost, and is not too boring. You may find that the cheapest way to an exercise machine is to join a local health club having the machine that you want to use. Even so, that will mean fitting into your day a stop at the health club at the proper time to use their machine. If you haven't time in your day for a brisk long walk, you probably won't be able to manage time for this stop either. You will then need to buy a machine, and they can be expensive. Adequate exercise machines are always expensive. The cheap ones are not worth it.

One answer is to buy a treadmill for running indoors. Good ones are expensive — about $1,000 — and they have all of the advantages and disadvantages of jogging and running: Since it is a weightbearing exercise you therefore expend more calories per minute doing the exercise; since it is a form of running it is a jarring type of exercise and can be rough on the joints. But it is indoors, in the comfort of your home, and especially appealing when it is storming outside.

Stationary bicycles are the best selling and most popular exercise machine. They are, compared to other machines, the least expensive. Since they are not weightbearing, you need to increase *duration* of exercise to achieve the same results you would with a weight-bearing exercise machine such as a treadmill or cross-country skiing machine. Stationary bikes can be tough on the back but if you are comfortable on one and will not allow it to gather dust, a stationary bicycle can be a good solution.

Rowing machines can also be difficult for people with low back pain, but rowing is an excellent form of aerobic exercise. Since it is nonweightbearing, you will need to work harder than you would with a weight-bearing form of exercise to achieve the same results.

The best exercise machine of all is a machine that simulates the best aerobic exercise of all, cross-country skiing. Cross-country skiing exercises the entire body in a way that other machines and other forms of aerobic exercise cannot. It is a jarless form of exercise even though weightbearing. It is therefore easy on the joints. Cross-country skiers consistently score higher on conditioning tests than any other class of athlete.

Let me tell you about one such skier .... All winter long, every winter, one hospital employee tears home from the hospital at 3:00 p.m. everyday to cross-country ski. He charges out his back door, across the snow and around his sauna, and off into the woods beyond. He shoots along the snow-covered tops of stone walls that cut through the woods, races down the logging roads over to the far pasture, then up a ridge, and, skating with his long nordic skis, he gathers up speed downhill to the lake. He races the length of the lake, and is soon back up through the woods, startling the jays, and back to his house in no time, finishing his fifteen mile loop, covered with sweat, and ready for some of his homemade beer. He is over fifty, looks thirty, and will undoubtedly live to be one of those old codgers you see rocking on their porches throwing stones at the cars from Massachusetts.

A cross-country ski simulator doesn't have the snow, or the woods, or the jays — but if you can't have all that, you can still have the exercise. NordicTrack (address in the bibliography) makes, according to Consumer Reports, the best cross-country ski simulator. Their machine is not cheap ... but on the other hand it's about the same price as a color television set. Make a choice. For my money, it is the best exercise machine available.

Exercise and Life   I have busied you with intensity and frequency and duration, with seconds and calories. But what I really have wanted to say was: Start simply, stay active, have fun with exercise. With activity and exercise, find your own golden mean. But *do start.* Some exercise is better than none at all. Make the decision that you are going to do it, and then get the medical clearance we talked about. Consider the medical checkup as a first step up the slope toward the ridge where the wild caraway grows. Decide for yourself that this is the most important step in your life. Decide that company and society and work and Little League and other people cannot get in the way of this because if this doesn't happen, if exercise does not become a part of your life, you may not be around for company and society and Little League and parties.

Neither should you become overly regimented. Be gentle with yourself, as the saying goes. Nevertheless, do not exercise only *when* you have the time, *make time* for your exercise. Put exercise before anything else, so that everything else will still have a part of you someday . . . . a better part of you.

Avoid the tendency to become rigid, the making of complicated schedules and charts, and the keeping of complicated records. If you are forced to use an exercise machine, you will find when you are on vacation and away you cannot take the machine with you. And what will you do then? Remember that exercise is part of the *form* of your life and remember that the *content* can differ. When you're on vacation you will have leisure time, time for that brisk, joyous walk that you have never had the time to do. Vacation can then become for you a time for more fulfilling exercise, rather than a time to overeat and consume conspicuously.

Eventually, this exercise *will* become a part of your life, whether you are lucky enough to run with the wind, forced to peddle away furiously on a stationary bicycle while listening to Mozart, or whether you slide away on your NordicTrack machine, dreaming that you are lucky enough to live in Maine.

What exercise will teach you, what you will find when you reach the top of the ridge, is how to trust yourself. That is the secret of self-esteem. Simply by making a plan for yourself, simply by improving yourself through fitness, you will gain the sense of self-sufficiency. You will know the power in your hips and in your shoulders, you will never panic when the float plane doesn't come, and someday you will find yourself sitting on the end of a dock in the night, hoping beyond hope that civilization will never come to your rescue.

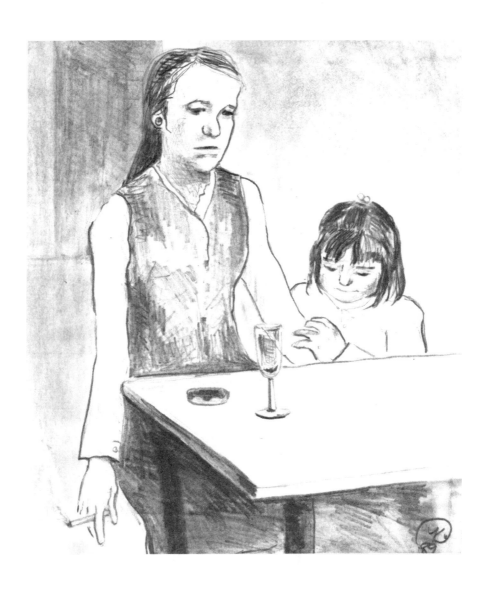

8

Tobacco and Alcohol

"If it weren't for cigarettes I'd be out of a job."

James C. Hanson, M.D.
Lung Specialist

SMOKING: A DANGEROUS JOURNEY

What a wonderful habit is cigarette smoking! It's not just a matter of having something to do with your hands. Cigarettes allow you to stand astride the top of a mountain in tight jeans, squinting at the sun. Cigarettes give you the role of the emancipated woman: slim, sexy, and so very cool. Cigarettes will let you fit in with the group: You can be like your dad, imitate your older brothers, and fit in with the crowd. And the good you do for the American economy with your smoking is incalculable. The tobacco industry is one of the top five industries in the United States. Because of government price supports and incentives for growing tobacco over the past fifty years, the tobacco farmer can make between $3,000 and $4,000 per acre. And you as a smoker have a part in this. And beyond the great taste and less tar, beyond the cool smoke and the jobs you create, beyond the boost to our gross national product, cigarettes can take you to some fascinating places.

Here is a story about one such fantastic voyage.... He found himself surrounded by the pristine sterility of stainless steel. From somewhere within this chamber, the electronic circuitry hummed about him. He checked the digital readouts on the monitors: The chronometer read 0540, temperature 37.3 degrees Centigrade, pulse interval 853 milliseconds. He scanned the red and gold diodes and the tracings of the oscilloscopes and rested his eyes on the tangle of tubing and wiring leading to and from the computer which controlled the various life support systems. Everything seemed to be functioning well. He checked all of the parameters. He found everything in order. Technicians noiselessly scurried in and out of this chamber with barely a glance at him. He felt as though he might be some all-powerful god to be served.

He marveled at this technological achievement. Everything seemed to be focused upon him, and yet he realized that the technology was in itself an end. It provided jobs, promoted research, and would ultimately be improved upon to support other anticipated flights. He marveled also at where he found himself in this moment. Although he was about to begin the greatest flight of his life, still he found himself insulated from all of the frantic preparation, separated by a vagueness that he couldn't quite penetrate. He wondered whether, when others had made similar trips, they had researched their destinations. Or did they feel as unprepared, as much on the edge of an abyss as he did at this moment? He realized now that it was too late for any further preparation. His feelings of expectation were tinged with regret. He would have preferred to feel more prepared.

Would he be aware of the journey itself? Would he sense the time change and the transition of matter to antimatter? Or would he simply find himself there? He didn't have any answers. There was no one to give them to him. Not all of the computers in the galaxy jammed with all of the microchips in the universe could plot his exact course.

One of the technicians smiled at him, nodded, and said something to him. However, he was focused elsewhere, and could only be dimly aware of her. She and all the surrounding instruments were peripheral to him. His anticipation consumed him. He was about to leave. Someone had said that he was too young to make the trip. But it did not matter now. He was waiting for the launch and at the same time wishing for more time to prepare.

His mind began to wander. He wondered if he had been premedicated for the liftoff. He couldn't recall if pre-flight drugs had been a part of the protocol. He became aware of the hemispheric dichotomy that was his brain. His left brain marveled at the irony of his daydreaming right cortex. He was amazed, with this great day here at last, with all of the circuitry and electronic gadgetry, that he could find himself wandering amid the memories of other years.

He recalled a hot summer day of long ago. He could feel the warmth of the orchard, the dappled sunlight under the trees, the camaraderie of his childhood friends. He was there with them! There were no budgets, no fiscal responsibilities, no computer printouts, no cares at all. He felt only the juvenile paranoia of the

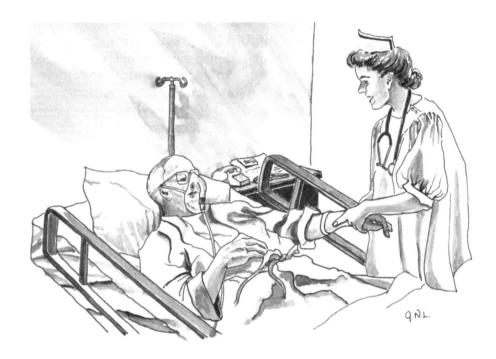

threat of the police, or some sneaky archbishop, suddenly sweeping down upon them to catch them all smoking cornsilk. The apple blossoms faded from his memory and dissolved, to be replaced by the trappings of the senior prom. The in-crowd swept him along to celebrate adulthood with Camels, Luckies, and beer. Two more decades drifted by.

"Launch time is approaching!" his left-brain screamed. He dreamed on. The irony! With the impending flight and the uncharted territory ahead, still he was immersed in memories of yesterday. And why did his thoughts focus on the cigarette? Here in this memory he squints through the tobacco's acrid smoke to line up a billiard shot. Now he savors the first drag of the morning. And there, at the finest restaurant in the city, he delights in the taste of tobacco with his coffee and dessert. In this scene he inhales a whole pack of cigarettes while his first child is born. And at his board meeting, his secretaries make certain his ashtray is at hand.

Another technician entered, interrupting his reverie, looking quite stern and grave. He was about to inquire about launch time. Then he decided to submit passively and simply let events happen. The technician left quickly. Discreet memories were replaced by waves of primitive emotion. Each surge of emotion, unrelated to external events, was quickly replaced by another emotion. First came sorrow, ponderous and slow. Next joy skipped in. Then came nagging regret, followed by anger, gesturing wildly. Courage and fear and elation and despair — each had its turn with him. He became aware that he was leaving. His journey had begun.

The chronometer ticked to 0541. At age 54, he had breathed his last. His doctor pronounced him dead.

Health Consequences of Smoking

Smokers exercise an incredible amount of denial about the risks of smoking, and, largely because of advertising, even non-smokers perceive the risks to be lower than they actually are. Though AIDS is a serious and frightening disease, nevertheless let's get some perspective from real numbers. From 1981 to the present, about 66,000 people in the United States have contracted AIDS. By 1992, there may be 300,000 more cases of AIDS. Now consider *only* the risk of lung cancer from cigarette smoking. Forget *all* of the other health consequences of smoking. Lung cancer directly attributed to cigarette smoking will kill 150,000 to 200,000 Americans every year. In addition, smoking is a major cause of coronary heart disease, which in turn is a leading cause of death. The earlier in life one begins smoking, the longer one smokes, and the more deeply one inhales, the greater is the risk of heart disease. Smoking causes high blood pressure, increasing the likelihood of heart disease. Those who smoke pipes and cigars are not free from risk either; their risk of developing heart disease is somewhere between that for nonsmokers and cigarette smokers. Smoking greatly increases the risk of sustaining a stroke as well as the risk of circulatory problems.

The 'Benefits' of Cigarette Smoking

- Lung cancer
- Cancer of the voice box
- Cancer of the bladder
- Cancer of the pancreas
- Cancer of the esophagus
- Cancer of the mouth and tongue
- Cancer of the stomach
- Emphysema
- Loss of income (sick days)
- Infant illnesses of smoking mothers
- Stained teeth
- Tobacco smell

Cancer is a major consequence of cigarette smoking. Yet knowledge of that fails to deter most smokers. Cancer always happens to someone else.

Some time ago I spoke to high school juniors and seniors about cigarette smoking. I had with me three of my patients: a man in his fifties whose lung cancer was removed surgically five years before, and who continues to sneak one or two cigarettes a month; a woman in her sixties tethered to an oxygen machine, who continually feels breathless, and carries her tank everywhere; and finally, a woman of thirty-five, a two pack a day smoker, who vowed that afternoon that she would quit. The last patient, the woman of thirty-five, continues to smoke to this day. Smoking is a very powerful addiction indeed — some researchers liken it to the addiction to heroin.

Few people actually witness the serious consequences of cigarette smoking. Those few patients of mine whom I have taken over to the hospital and whom I have introduced to a patient dying from emphysema, for example, those few patients have had great success in quitting smoking. In the main, however, hospitalized patients dying of cancer, emphysema, or heart disease, all consequences of cigarette smoking, are kept out of view, their lessons unavailable to the committed smoker. Smoking causes, in so many and such devious ways, prolonged and horrible discomfort. Smoking is not simply a longevity issue. *It is pain and suffering.*

Here is a statistic that may cause you to get out your calculator:

An average of five and a half minutes of life is lost for each cigarette smoked.

Smoking has many risks; the overall death rate for smokers is seventy percent greater than for nonsmokers. And in pregnancy, for example, women who smoke give birth to smaller babies and increase their baby's risk of death. Women who smoke and use birth control pills have an increased risk of stroke, blood clots, and heart attacks. But the greatest danger of all, in my estimation, is that smokers teach young people how to smoke.

A Smoker's Legacy

A wake is a heavy affair even when the deceased is seventy years old. Men, especially, seem nervous about attending such things. They need a break from the grieving. Fortunately for us, in the back of the funeral home there was an oasis removed from the black crepe: the smoking room. Each well-stuffed chair had its ornate ashtray. The smell of tobacco and the blue-gray haze was comforting to all of us. We lit up, took long slow drags, and began to relax. We, the men of the family, reunited for this one day of grieving, were joined together as well in this ritual of manhood. I could look around the room and see the faces of my brothers, cousins, and uncles soften, their moods become placid. Smoking relaxed us. We began to reminisce. We recalled other, happier family reunions. We talked about the good old days, the holidays and special times, the turkey dinners, sledding, and closeness of family.

In those days, as kids, we'd stamp off the snow, run inside to the warmth of our grandfather's home, waist high to everyone. Dodging the wet kisses and hugs, we'd settle in the living room and begin building houses and roads using the dozens of his cigarette packages as building blocks. My cousins and I would watch the men and store away their gestures, their laughs, and phrases, to use later on. The women clattered dishes in the kitchen as each man, holding a can of beer and a cigarette in one hand, as only a man can do, laughed and teased each other. The patriarch of the family would yell "Tidbits!" and we would run for the kitchen and for the carving of the turkey. His cigarette dangling, his left eye squinting against the smoke, he'd pass out bits of warm turkey and skin to his "little chickens." Each of us, busy with studying the lessons of manhood, watched his every move.

At dinner the lessons continued. Uncles rolled their eyes and aunts were politely quiet, as we learned about doing things well and loving our family and how to raise the best turkeys and how not to smoke until we were twenty-one. Each boy at the table learned his lessons well.

With the table cleared, the women gossiped in the kitchen and the men sat down to poker. We watched, fascinated, in the living room and tried to imitate with games of our own. The patriarch always seemed to win. And all of the men continually nursed lighted cigarettes throughout the game.

With advancing age, time becomes more important than material assets for anyone. With the family patriarch's retirement now a reality, he gained time. But this time for him was less than it might have been. The family called it simply old age, but his pursed lips, barrel chest, and slow measured steps were more than the result of old age. "No wind" he said and gave up his garden, his roses, and his hens. Deprived of air, he gave up driving, then short walks in the fall, then even going out of doors. The vigorous, tatooed old sailor became a shut-in. He lived his threescore and ten, yet surrendered his golden years. And he left a legacy, a dark inheritance for all of his grandchildren. His grandsons, every one, learned to smoke.

In the funeral parlor's smoking room, my cousin,

seventeen and confused with all this death and sadness, snubs out his third cigarette and moves away to be with his mother. The rest of us take a quick long last drag and follow him out. Great Uncle Henry, brother of the deceased, looking more like sixty than eighty, is a haunting example of what his brother might have been. He rushes about, greeting and comforting everyone, marveling at how we have grown. He has the wind to do it. He has never smoked. But no one there makes the connection. And no one can see himself in the casket.

Our human nature often prevents our learning from the simplest lessons life has to give. We forget how precious is our health, how precious is the quality of life. And we all lose the notion of the power of our actions, *actions studied carefully by our children,* for whom words alone are never enough.

Kicking the Habit

It pays to quit smoking. On that, all experts agree. Almost immediately, the risk of cancers and of heart disease begins decreasing. The risk of developing emphysema, especially if one quits before symptoms develop, also decreases, approaching the risk for a nonsmoker. But it is hard to quit smoking cigarettes. The addiction is frighteningly powerful. There are really two addictions: the **psychological habit** of smoking, and the **chemical dependence** upon nicotine.

How do you treat such a powerful addiction? How can you reasonably expect to quit smoking? First, it helps a great deal if a physician tells you to quit. Surprisingly few physicians do that. Yet such advice from a physician markedly increases the chances of success. Next, make sure your spouse also quits smoking; it is nearly impossible to quit smoking if someone else in the house continues to smoke. Now, enlist the help of self-help groups, fashioned after that most successful of all such groups, Alcoholics Anonymous. Almost every community has some sort of no smoking clinic, class, or self-help group; often such clinics meet at the time of the Great American Smokeout every fall.

Now pick a target date when you will quit smoking completely. 'Cold-turkey' is better than cutting down.

Gradually tapering off cigarettes just does not work as well. It is very helpful if the target date for quitting is at the beginning of a vacation of a week or more. A vacation can mean withdrawing yourself from everything that you associate with smoking. Breaking those associations is very important to quitting. On vacation you are away from the "smoke-break," the coffee break, the stresses of the work place, the demands of the family — you are on a vacation from the stress you use cigarettes to relieve.

You will be more successful if you give up those associations you link with smoking. You must plan to give them up, at least for a while. Select yours from the following list.

Favorite Companions of Smokers

- A beer and a cigarette
- Working under pressure and a cigarette
- Coffee and a cigarette
- Being with others who smoke
- Sitting at the table after dinner and a cigarette
- Arguing with your spouse and a cigarette
- Playing cards and a cigarette
- A cocktail and a cigarette
- Feeling lonely and a cigarette
- TV and a cigarette
- Talking on the telephone and a cigarette
- Your favorite chair and a cigarette
- Reading the morning paper and a cigarette
- A short drive and a cigarette
- Waiting for service in a restaurant and a cigarette
- A long drive and a cigarette

It may be helpful to see your doctor just before the target date. It's human nature to forget one's New Year's resolutions before February. At this final meeting with your doctor before the target date, review with him or her the hazards of cigarette smoking, the health consequences of quitting, your reasons for quitting, and the economic consequences of doing so. (With regard to the latter, the money you save from quitting smoking will purchase that exercise machine!)

Because the addiction to cigarettes is really both psychological and chemical, consider using a nicotine-containing chewing gum. This will increase your chances of success, because you can cope first with the withdrawal from the psychological habit of smoking, and contend later with the chemical dependence on nicotine, withdrawing from the nicotine-gum three to six months after you quit cigarettes. Be advised that nicotine-gum will not cause you to want to quit. The gum will not make you enjoy quitting smoking. But it will make it easier to quit.

The first week of quitting is pure hell. See your doctor toward the end of that first week. You will need the support and it will improve your chances of success. Remember that quitting smoking is one of the hardest things anyone can do; you need all the help and support you can muster. Plan to see your doctor frequently after that, especially if you have no support from a self-help group.

As the weeks go on, the quitting becomes easier but you will still be struck suddenly by that tremendous urge to reach for the cigarettes. The urges are natural and tend to occur around the associations we have talked about above. Physicians who smoke seem to have an easier time quitting. I think that this is because they *are* continually reminded of the terrible nature of the diseases caused by smoking. So it was with me when I quit smoking twenty years ago.

Here is how it happened . . . . When you are a new doctor it is as though you are newly in love. Everything about medicine is exciting, enchanting. You embrace all of your professional existence with everything you have, unafraid, unaware of your own vulnerability, as yet unburned by death and loss — without caution. One of my first patients as an intern was a man whom I called Pat. I loved him dearly: I hadn't yet learned that patients die and that doctors should love with caution. It was from Pat that I learned where the trout were, and which flies they would take. We had two things in common: trout fishing and smoking.

Pat's initial routine chest x-ray was horrible: A huge cancer lay within the arch of the largest of arteries in the body, the aorta. The only blessing in this was that Pat would die suddenly.

As do all young doctors, I wrestled with whether to tell him that he had an incurable cancer and that his days were numbered. In the end I did, and, as are most patients in that situation, Pat was grateful to know. His edges softened, he relaxed, and *he* began to console *me*. He could sense my own grief. He said that he had only one fear. He was afraid that he would die in his apartment, that no one would find him, and that he would lie there for days. That thought bothered him. I promised him that I would call him every night before I left the hospital. For four months, each night I would call him, the phone would ring once and Pat would pick it up and say, "I'm fine boy. Thanks."

On the day he didn't answer. I threw away my cigarettes.

Breaking the addiction to cigarettes is very difficult. Relapses occur. Treat those relapses in yourself and in others gently. *And keep trying.*

ALCOHOLISM   **In Another Land.** Geographical isolation is conducive to intermarriage. In some cantons of Switzerland, in certain regions of the Himalayas, and even in certain areas of rural America, marriage between close relatives is common. Where this occurs, there will be increased numbers of inherited, or genetic, diseases.

Most genetic diseases require two doses of an abnormal gene to manifest the disease. Since such abnormal genes may run in families, offspring of intermarriages are more likely to have two doses of the abnormal gene. Consider the classical example of the disease **phenylketonuria.** Through the inherited lack of a simple genetic message, a child may be born without the proper amount of one particular chemical

— a chemical so essential that, lacking it, the child will become severely retarded and require institutionalization. Because of the lack of this single chemical, the afflicted child cannot process a simple amino acid, phenylalanine, which is found in the normal diet. The treatment for such a child is simple: Eliminate phenylalanine from the child's diet, and he or she will be a normal healthy human being. But if you, from ignorance, continue to feed the child phenylalanine, you will be left with a mentally deficient patient with an IQ of less than 50, requiring constant care for the rest of his or her life.

Now imagine a land where geographical isolation has led to a modest amount of intermarriage of first and second cousins. And in this imagined land, such intermarriage has led to the appearance of one particular genetic disease. For the sake of our discussion, we will consider the disease to be biochemical in basis, but far more complicated than the example given with phenylketonuria.

And let us neither focus on how the disease is inherited nor on what its biochemistry may be, but rather on how the people of this imagined country *view* this genetic disease, and what they *do* about it. We shall say that the disease itself is prevalent. Because of the geographic isolation, the intermarriage, and the disease's inheritance patterns, one in twenty of this country's population are afflicted with this inherited disease. Untreated, the disease exacts a terrible price. It attacks the brain in the centers of motion and coordination. It destroys the higher centers of the brain, the centers for creativity, for memory, and for emotion. It causes cancer, heart failure, and internal bleeding and, in severe cases, invariably results in early death.

Our imagined society is not ignorant of the disease's mechanisms. They are surrounded by the disease and know, to a person, that the disease is caused by a simple chemical in the diet, just as phenylalanine in the diet destroys the brain of the phenylketonuric. Yet, this society behaves in an odd way towards its people suffering from the genetic disease. For one thing, the people of our imagined country view the problem not as a disease at all, but rather as a moral problem. Those afflicted are branded as morally bankrupt, constitutionally weak, and, more simply, they are looked upon as baser elements of society. The media portrays the disease as comical. Those afflicted are made fun of — portrayed as clowns. Their nervous system symptoms are painted in ridiculous caricatures. People laugh at them, point to them, step over them in the streets when they have reached near-death. They are scarcely regarded.

Amazingly, the disease is glamorized on television in this imagined land. To have the disease may be a mark of success. And in this way the disease can actually be promoted. Or, those affected may be fired from their jobs because of the disease. And the country's doctors underdiagnose the disease because most of them also believe that the disease is more a matter of morality than genetics, and because the physicians prefer not to take care of these people. They would rather keep busy with other patients having more "interesting" problems.

In this far off land, the offending chemical in the diet is known: Its chemical structure is more simple than the amino acid phenylalanine. Nevertheless, consumption of the chemical is promoted by society. The chemical is often included in foods and in cooking without warning. The chemical is sold on every corner, in every supermarket, and in every grocery store in the land.

Our imagined country gives us a grand example of national schizophrenia: Those with the disease are scorned, ridiculed, and disenfranchised from society. But consuming the chemical is glorified, promoted by people of the stature of an Olympic athlete, a movie star, a successful businessman.

Cut off from the mainstream of society, misunderstood by their friends and neighbors, those with the disease meet secretly, anonymously, as did Christians in their catacombs. They try to help themselves, as no one else in society is willing to do it.

And now you have a true picture of alcoholism in America.

We know about our prejudices: the drunken Irish, the drunken Indian, the drunken nigger. We can see them if we will only look, and we know that we don't *want* to look, don't *want* to see them. We find it hard to consider this a disease, we don't want to care *about* them, and we don't want to care *for* them. We know about alcohol's terrible price: the fractured families, the abuse, the deaths in drunkenness, from drunkenness. And still we sell it in every corner store, extol its virtues on television, and radio, in the glossy magazines, for all our children to hear and read. We despise the weakness alcohol represents to us, and promote the disease alcoholism.

Nor do all of the problems related to alcohol rest with alcoholics. Most alcohol-related automobile accidents do not involve "alcoholics." What about family violence, family financial problems, and teenage death on graduation night?

A Difficult Diagnosis

Why is alcoholism so difficult to diagnose? Alcoholics exercise a great deal of denial. They deny their disease, in part because of social condemnation and fear of moral judgment, and seldom give an accurate history of alcohol consumption and problems resulting from it. The physician has to dig for this information. The alcoholic has to be pressed for an accurate history. But because of their own attitudes and values, physicians do not do this well. Some physicians view the alcoholic as being weak of moral fiber, self-destructive, and too hopeless to be helped. And because physicians know that alcoholics can be difficult patients to care for, physicians have a subliminal resistance to making the diagnosis. Why make the day more difficult by diagnosing an alcoholic? Communication is jeopardized further by the alcoholic's denial and by the whole range of emotion presented by the alcoholic, emotions of anger, hostility, and self-deprecation.

Physicians in training receive very little teaching about alcoholism or about how to diagnose and treat it.

Instead, society's attitudes about alcoholics and alcoholism are reinforced in medical school. Young doctors in training are taught to view the drunk with disdain.

Alcoholism is a complex disease of complex causes and protean manifestations. Unlike phenylketonuria, alcoholism does not fit into a neat paragraph in a textbook. It is, as diseases go, today's "great masquerader," as was syphilis fifty years ago. Alcoholism presents itself in so many forms, with so many signs and symptoms, that only the well-trained physician looking for the disease will consistently make the diagnosis. The first and hardest step in diagnosis is to suspect alcoholism. Simple questionnaires (Tables 8-1 and 8-2), when approached honestly by patients and doctors, have a high degree of reliability for making the diagnosis.

A Study in Complexity

Alcoholism is best thought of as a mosaic of many diseases: a mixed population of patients unable to contend with alcohol, having their lives disrupted by it because of genetic, biochemical, environmental, or psychological reasons, or because of a combination of these factors. And it is because of these factors, however they interplay, that the alcoholic cannot control consumption of alcohol.

Because it completely dissolves in water, alcohol can travel anywhere in the body that water also goes, that is, virtually to every living tissue. And because in certain concentrations alcohol is toxic to living tissue, every cell in the body can be subject to that toxicity. Because alcohol is a good solvent for other chemicals, some of which are known to be cancer-causing, consumption of alcohol may increase the alcoholic's exposure to carcinogens. And because alcohol has empty calories without any value for nutrition, when consumed in excess alcohol depresses appetite, leading to the malnutrition we so frequently see in the heavy drinker.

Because alcohol is so toxic and can travel to any tissue in the body, its toxic effects can destroy the liver, pancreas, intestines, and heart muscle. Alcohol regularly causes sexual impotence and is associated with cancers

TABLE 8–1   Michigan Alcoholism Screening Test (MAST)

Questions	Circle One	
1. Do you feel you are a normal drinker?	Yes (0)	No (2)
2. Do friends or relatives think you are a normal drinker?	Yes (0)	No (2)
3. Have you ever attended a meeting of Alcoholics Anonymous (AA)?	Yes (5)	No (0)
4. Have you ever lost friends or girlfriends or boyfriends because of drinking?	Yes (2)	No (0)
5. Have you ever gotten into trouble at work because of drinking?	Yes (2)	No (0)
6. Have you ever neglected your obligations, your family, or your work for two or more days in a row because you were drinking?	Yes (2)	No (0)
7. Have you ever had delirium tremens or severe shaking, heard voices, or seen things that were not there after heavy drinking?	Yes (2)	No (0)
8. Have you ever gone to anyone for help about your drinking?	Yes (5)	No (0)
9. Have you ever been in a hospital because of drinking?	Yes (5)	No (0)
10. Have you ever been arrested for drunk driving or driving after drinking?	Yes (2)	No (0)

A score greater than five indicates alcoholism. Scores are arrived at by adding up the values for answers.

TABLE 8–2   CAGE Questionnaire For Diagnosing Alcoholism

1. Have you ever felt you should Cut down on your drinking?

2. Have people Annoyed you by criticizing your drinking?

3. Have you ever felt Guilty about your drinking?

4. Have you ever had to have an Eye-opener, a drink first thing in the morning, to steady your nerves or get rid of a hangover?

Two yeses suggest alcoholism and three or more are diagnostic of alcoholism.

of the liver, esophagus, and mouth. We see evidence everyday of alcohol's effect on the central nervous system: a regular, predictable atrophying of the brain, producing significant cognitive impairment and extreme problems of coordination. *A proper listing of alcoholism's effect on the body would in fact require pages to list.*

Misconceptions persist. A frequently held belief is that one must be falling-down drunk in order to suffer the ravages of alcohol. Nothing is further from the truth. Because the alcoholic becomes tolerant to the intoxicating effects of alcohol, the alcoholic can consume large quantities, even toxic quantities, of the drug without in the least appearing incapacitated.

Treatment of Alcoholism

Seventy percent of alcoholics can be cured. This is a better cure rate than for most forms of cancer, and far better certainly than the cure rate for obesity. The main stumbling blocks to cure are two: the physician's reluctance to make the diagnosis, and the patient's reluctance to admit the problem. When these blocks to the diagnosis, together with other impediments (the family "enabler" and society's condemnation of the patient, for example) are removed, treatment may be extremely effective. Here is what I have come to rely upon for treatment.

In my experience, any alcoholic who joins **Alcoholics Anonymous** has a high rate of success for beating the disease. Alcoholics Anonymous' basic tenets are outlined in Tables 8-3 and 8-4. The organization is independent, has no building or superstructure, no federal funding, no political, social, or medical agendas other than helping its members. But it works. Alcoholics Anonymous is free. Its members are as diverse as is the population afflicted with the disease. So strongly do I believe in AA for the alcoholic, that I strongly encourage that any alcoholic patient of mine join AA even if he or she has gone through a twenty-eight day treatment program, has a psychologist or psychiatrist, and *no matter how firmly the alcoholic believes that he or she is "cured."*

I do not believe in "controlled drinking." In the Seventies, the Rand Corporation released a study which alleged that alcoholics, after being "treated" for their disease, could re-enter society and continue to

TABLE 8-3 Alcoholics Anonymous—The Twelve Steps

 1. We admitted we were powerless over alcohol, that our lives had become unmanageable.
 2. Came to believe that a Power greater than ourselves could restore us to sanity.
 3. Made a decision to turn our will and our lives over to the care of God *as we understood Him.*
 4. Made a searching and fearless moral inventory of ourselves.
 5. Admitted to God, to ourselves and to another human being the exact nature of our wrongs.
 6. Were entirely ready to have God remove all these defects of character.
 7. Humbly asked Him to remove our shortcomings.
 8. Made a list of all persons we had harmed, and became willing to make amends to them all.
 9. Made direct amends to such people wherever possible, except when to do so would injure them or others.
10. Continued to take personal inventory, and when we were wrong, promptly admitted it.
11. Sought through prayer and meditation to improve our conscious contact with God, *as we understood Him,* praying only for knowledge of His will for us and the power to carry that out.
12. Having had a spiritual awakening as the result of these Steps, we tried to carry this message to alcoholics, and to practice these principles in all our affairs.

drink in a controlled fashion. In my experience, and in the experience of others, this has not and will not work.

Antabuse is another form of treatment for alcoholism. Antabuse, the drug trade name for disulfiram, interferes with the body's metabolism of alcohol. An alcoholic taking Antabuse gets violently ill after ingesting even small amounts of alcohol. In theory Antabuse is a great idea, but in practice it has a limited role. I rarely prescribe it and tend to rely more upon AA.

Treating an alcoholic also means treating the alcoholic's family. Failure to do so neglects optimum treatment of the alcoholic. **Al-Anon** provides the kind of support and advice for spouses of alcoholics that Alcoholics Anonymous provides for the patient. Al-

TABLE 8–4   The Twelve Traditions of Alcoholics Anonymous

1. Our common welfare should come first; personal recovery depends upon AA unity.
2. For our group purpose there is but one ultimate authority — a loving God as He may express Himself in our group conscience. Our leaders are but trusted servants; they do not govern.
3. The only requirement for AA membership is a desire to stop drinking.
4. Each group should be autonomous except in matters affecting other groups or AA as a whole.
5. Each group has but one primary purpose — to carry out its message to the alcoholic who still suffers.
6. An AA group ought never endorse, finance, or lend the AA name to any related facility or outside enterprise, lest problems of money, property, and prestige divert us from our primary purpose.
7. Every AA group ought to be fully self-supporting, declining outside contributions.
8. Alcoholics Anonymous should remain forever nonprofessional, but our service centers may employ special workers.
9. AA, as such, ought never to be organized, but we may create service boards or committees directly responsible to those they serve.
10. Alcoholics Anonymous has no opinion on outside issues; hence the AA name ought never be drawn into public controversy.
11. Our public relations policy is based on attraction rather than promotion; we need always maintain personal anonymity at the level of press, radio, and films.
12. Anonymity is the spiritual foundation of our Traditions, ever reminding us to place principles before personalities.

Ateen provides similar guidance for teenagers whose parents are alcoholics.

Four Alcoholics   A patient of mine owns a very successful business. She is an attractive middle-aged woman, very intelligent and very capable of expressing herself. I had been seeing her for three or four years for problems of high blood pressure and for a tendency toward gout. Because she was so sophisticated, it never occurred to me that her hypertension and problem with gout might be caused by alcoholism. She seemed always well-nourished, neat, trim, and in control of herself. But one of the advantages of practicing in a small town is that sometimes you obtain helpful information about your patients from other sources. My patient's brother was also a patient of mine. One day during his office visit he said to me, "Look Doctor, I'm probably overstepping my bounds but I have to tell you this. My sister is a patient of yours and I think she has a problem. She keeps a bottle at her office, in her desk drawer. She goes through a fifth a day. Nobody else knows this, not her husband, nobody. I thought you ought to know."

I used this information to get through to my patient by way of a back door. I simply told her that, in some cases, high blood pressure and gout can be caused by too much alcohol. Did she consume a lot of alcohol I asked?

"Well," she said, "I do drink."

I asked her how much and she said "regularly" and I said what does "regularly" mean and she said "well, everyday" and I said "well, how much everyday" and we went on like this. That's the way it usually goes. In the end we got to the facts. I told her that if she was going through a fifth of Vodka everyday then she was probably an alcoholic. This shocked her. She used alcohol to get through a very tense, stressful day in the fast lane. She had no idea that she might be an alcoholic. Neither did her husband. Once confronted with her problem and able to see it, she went willingly to an alcohol-rehabilitation center. After twenty-eight days of inpatient treatment there, she joined, and still belongs to, Alcoholics Anonymous. She has been abstinent for eighteen months. I have every hope that she will continue alcohol-free.

A second patient was a much more "obvious" alcoholic. He presented to me about five years ago in the emergency room with massive internal bleeding, a terribly scarred liver, and a swollen abdomen: the hallmarks of the severely diseased alcoholic. He *knew* that he had a problem with alcohol. He knew that his broken marriage and abused, resentful, angry children had been the result of alcoholism. Miraculously, he survived his acute illness of five years ago. It was the experience of that illness which caused him, I think, to see what he was doing to himself. He had neither the money nor the insurance to cover the cost of a prolonged inpatient rehabilitation program. But Alcoholics Anonymous is free, and he joined. He attended meetings six nights a week. He still attends AA meetings, has abstained for five years, has had no further episodes of bleeding, and still comes to the office every six months to tease me about being "thirsty."

A third patient drank because his wife was an alcoholic. He drank because she drank and because "that's what one does in a university society." In an insidious way he too became an alcoholic, developed chronic pancreatitis, and came close to death. Ten years ago we debated whether to remove his inflamed pancreas. Because of his own firm conviction that he would no longer drink, we decided against the surgery. He has done very well these past ten years, because he has recognized his problem and because he regularly participates in Alcoholics Anonymous.

The last patient has not been so successful. One of the most brilliant, most intelligent patients I have had the good fortune to care for, this man has had periodic relapses every six months or so. He has been an alcoholic since his military days, when the quality of an officer was measured by how well he could hold his drink. Receptions, cocktail parties, 'happy hours,' low priced booze at the commissary, and free drinks wherever one turned were all a part of military life. How can one be a soldier and not be a two-fisted drinker? How can you be a man if you can't drink with the next guy? Can you be a good officer and not be seen at the officer's club? You cannot get promoted when all you drink is tonic water. Through an unusual complication of alcohol — destruction of his hip joints caused by the alcohol —this patient left the military with a total disability. Without a job, without an identity, and with very little self-esteem, his reasons for drinking became more than just those of acting the good soldier.

He has tried Antabuse without success. Because of

his intelligence and his adroitness at manipulation, he can defeat most psychiatrists. He continues to scorn Alcoholics Anonymous as "a bunch of skid row bums," "a hyper-religious organization of Jesus freaks," and "an addiction as terrible as alcohol itself." Those are in fact the common excuses one uses to avoid AA. *But they are weak excuses.*

Still he struggles with his disease and for eleven months out of the year he is abstinent. And he knows, when he has a relapse, he can call his doctor and get help without any moral judgments. And that is all we should offer anyone suffering from disease.

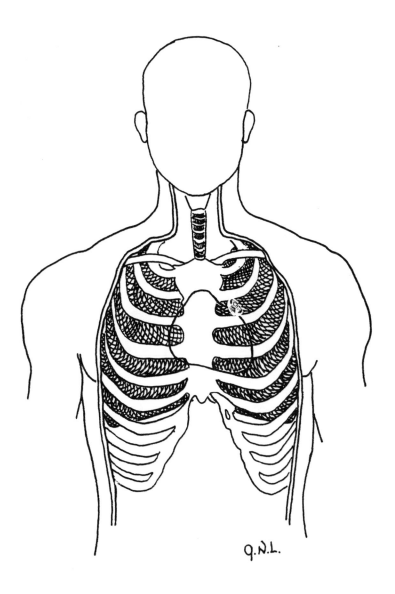

9

A Healthy Heart

Better to hunt in fields for health unbought,
Than fee the doctor for a nauseous drought.
The wise, for cure, on exercise depend;
God never made his work for man to mend.

John Dryden

After age ninety heart disease is God's fault.
Before age ninety, it's our fault.

Paul Dudley White

You know how it happens. You toss the football with the kids on the weekend and call it exercise. You have sporadic checks on your blood pressure — in a drug store, in the corridors of a shopping mall, at the time of your "annual" physical examination five years ago. You are dimly aware that your blood pressure tends to be high. You choose to ignore it, hoping the problem will go away. You pledge, again and again, to control your weight, watch what you eat, and decrease your salt consumption. Still, there is that doughnut staring at you and you are hungry. There are social obligations with their drinks and buffets, the family get-togethers where you are *expected* to eat, the evenings out, where one simply doesn't diet. Too soon you are fat, fifty, and out of shape — pinned to a bed in some intensive care unit, with electrodes on your chest, sweating your way through a heart attack, filled with regret. It happens every day.

In this chapter we shall examine heart disease and high blood pressure, and more specifically, *coronary artery disease* and its complications. When the layperson talks about a "heart attack" that may mean any problem relating to the heart: damage or infection of the heart valves, problems of heart rhythm and beating, or pain from, and damage to, the heart muscle because of coronary artery disease. In this chapter we will examine only the last of these heart problems, the how and why the arteries which supply blood and oxygen to the heart become damaged, and what problems occur because of that damage.

THE HEART: A PROPERLY TIMED PUMP

To understand what a "heart attack" is in a medical sense we need to understand how the heart works, and how fragile is its blood supply. Look at Figure 9-1. This is a cross-sectional view of the heart showing the major blood vessels entering and exiting the various chambers of the heart. For purposes of our present discussion, understand that the heart is a muscular pump, with the muscles squeezing blood out of its chambers through a series of one-way valves to the various parts of the body. The arrow designated "1" shows a cross-section of part

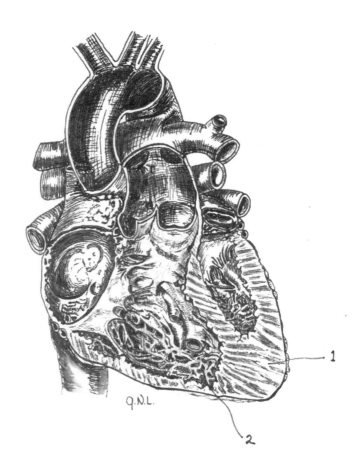

FIGURE 9-1   Cross-Sectional View of the Heart

of the heart muscle. The arrow designated "2" shows one of the internal chambers — in this case, the right ventricle. Because there are four chambers and four sets of valves, effective pumping depends upon a coordinated timing or **rhythmicity.** Because there is a considerable amount of tissue to be supplied with blood, oxygenated blood, coordinated effort of contraction of this muscle is also required. If the timing is lost, if the coordinated effort of contraction is lost, pumping will not be effective.

Consider your automobile, in which a simple rubber belt, the timing belt, coordinates the various openings and closings of the valves and apertures in the automobile's engine. The timing of these cycles is matched to the firing of the spark plug and the explosion inside the engine's pistons. If damage occurs to the timing belt, if part of its ridges are worn, or if part of it gets torn away, the engine's timing will be off. The piston may fire, for example, when there isn't any gasoline injected into the cylinder — such malfunction of timing will leave you stalled at the side of the road. If the timing is off only slightly, the pistons may not fire in a coordinated effort and the engine runs on one cylinder rather than six, which means that your automobile will hardly run at all.

Let us sum up this heart-automobile engine analogy: The worst thing that can happen to you, if you are desperately heading home, is for your automobile engine to stop utterly. The corresponding analogy is obvious: A problem of timing, rhythmicity, and coordinated effort of heart muscle can result in your heart's stopping, utterly.

That is the worst that can happen: that your automobile engine, or your heart, stops completely. But what if only a small part of the engine, one piston for example, or only one small part of your heart, is damaged? What then?

An automobile can run on three cylinders, and an airplane on one engine, although both do so with far less power and with considerably more danger. The same analogy holds true for the injured heart. If a portion of the muscle is damaged, assuming that the timing is not damaged, the heart can continue to pump, although less efficiently and with considerably less power.

Some Simple Anatomy

For simplicity's sake, let us assume that only one of the following can happen with your car: The timing belt snaps and you are stuck at the side of the road, or one piston stops firing and you can continue to motor along under decreased power. With respect to the anatomy of your heart, how do similar "breakdowns" occur?

Examine the two views of the heart as seen in Figure 9-2. These illustrations depict the heart from the front view and from the rear view. On the surface of the heart muscle are the **coronary arteries,** the three main arteries which together with their branches supply the pumping muscle with blood, nutrients, and oxygen.

In Figure 9-2, the three main coronary arteries are indicated by the numbers 3, 4, and 5. Note several

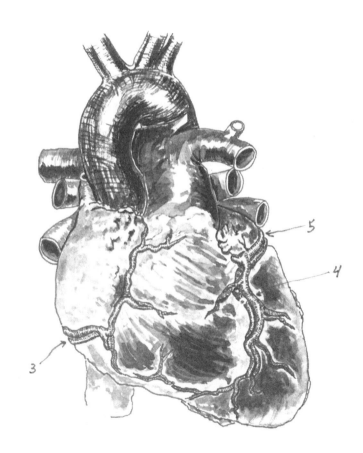

FIGURE 9–2A   Front View of the Heart

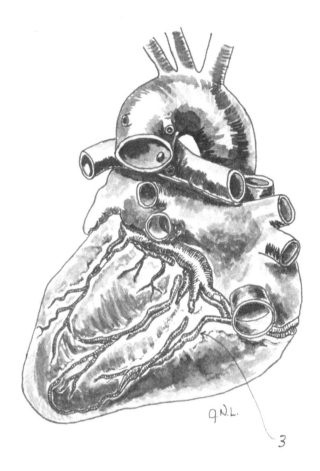

FIGURE 9–2B   Rear View of the Heart

important points about this anatomy:

- The arteries are on the outer surface of the heart, and so are easily accessible to the surgeon.
- There are only three arteries.
- The arteries are quite small in proportion to the importance of the job they perform.
- There is no "backup system," that is, each portion of the heart muscle seems to be supplied by only one branch of one artery.

Case Studies: Exceptions to The Rules

I have a patient-friend who is an exception to the "rules" discussed above in our engine analogy. He's an avid fly-fisherman and for most of his life has hiked through miles of woods and puckerbrush to cast a line on the surface of some unspoiled pond. Regularly, he makes the climb to Speck Pond, a mountain lake the hike to which would discourage a person half his age. When he isn't fishing, when he has to work in other words, his work has been in the woods, felling, limbing, and trucking wood to the mills of Maine. When this man suffered a heart attack, the amount of damaged muscle was small. His coronary circulation, the blood supply to his heart muscle, contained an extraordinary number of collaterals. These **collateral arteries,** back-up arteries, side-systems and detours, provided an extensive network of nourishment to his heart muscle. Hence, when one of his main coronary arteries became plugged, several alternate routes provided the threatened heart muscle with blood supply. His intense physical life had promoted the development of such a backup system. Such collaterals develop with strenuous exercise, but how frequently they do is not known.

When cholesterol builds up on the inner surfaces of a coronary artery, as crust deposits inside a pipe, physicians call that process "coronary artery disease." The deposits are called **plaques.** When the deposits reach a critical level, the flow of blood through the thickened crust is reduced to a trickle. The blood may suddenly clot. When that occurs, called **coronary thrombosis,** the blood supply to a portion of heart muscle is interrupted. That event, a "coronary event," can give rise to either or both of our "engine problems," as discussed above. The clot may form, interrupt the heart muscle's blood supply, and then dissolve of and by itself with the blood supply to the muscle restored, with the muscle spared, but with the timing mechanism interrupted for a few critical, and often fatal, seconds. In this type of heart attack, it doesn't matter whether the pistons and pumping action are normal and preserved; if the timing and rhythmicity are interrupted even for a few seconds, the pump functions improperly, and the brain dies.

Twenty years ago at the time of my hospital training, we had a patient with profound problems of heart rhythmicity. This patient, J. G., had a very faulty timing belt indeed. Someone counted up the number of times J. G. had been administered countershock to his chest because of problems in rhythmicity. The count totaled 800. At that time, in the 1960's, we had only a few drugs to offer J. G. for his problems of rhythmicity. For him, none of these drugs were effective. Ultimately, he died of his disease. Today, twenty years later, in addition to the plethora of new drugs available to treat problems of rhythm, surgery can actually be performed to correct the faulty timing belt. Alternatively, a small, pacemaker-like implantable electronic device can detect the rhythm problems when they occur and administer a slight shock from within the heart to correct the rhythm disturbance.

Suppose that the trickle of blood through a cholesterol **plaque** slows, clots, and solidifies. Suppose it does not dissolve by itself, that no therapy is initiated to dissolve it. And suppose that this coronary event does *not* interrupt heart rhythmicity. In this case, a portion of the heart muscle, deprived of its blood supply, may be injured permanently, ultimately to be replaced by scar tissue. Physicians term this a **myocardial infarction.** In this, the second of our engine problems, the heart patient runs on three cylinders.

Before we discuss additional actual patients, there is one other coronary event to understand. This we call **angina pectoris.**

Suppose that one or more of the coronary arteries is severely diseased with cholesterol deposits. One of these deposits blocks ninety percent of the internal diameter of one of the coronary arteries. Still, enough blood flows through the narrowed aperture to supply its heart muscle for ordinary everyday demands, demands such as driving to work, signing reports, and reading the evening paper. But other demands cause the heart muscle to pump more forcefully: demands such as the

Internal Revenue Service, the first heavy snowfall, or an argument with your spouse. Now, with this increased demand, the heart muscle does not get blood sufficient to meet the demand. Heart muscle receiving insufficient blood circulation, and yet not permanently damaged, suffers from **ischemia.** This ischemia, this insufficient blood supply for the work demanded of the heart muscle, gives rise to heart pain which we term **angina pectoris.**

To Summarize:

- The heart may suddenly stop because of a problem of timing or rhythmicity.
- The heart may pump less efficiently because a portion of muscle is damaged, but life goes on.
- Permanent damage to heart muscle is termed myocardial infarction.
- Insufficient blood supply to heart muscle for the work demanded of it is called ischemia.
- Both ischemia and infarction may give rise to various types of pain in varying intensity, or in fact no pain at all.
- The pain of ischemia we term angina pectoris. The term implies temporary rather than permanent heart muscle impairment.
- The pain of permanent injury, that is of myocardial infarction, may be of the same character as angina pectoris, although usually more severe and longer lasting.
- Ischemia of heart muscle, myocardial infarction, angina pectoris, and rhythm disturbances or problems of timing, may all result from coronary artery disease.
- Coronary artery disease results when cholesterol deposits inside the coronary arteries of the heart decrease the flow of blood through the arteries.

To illustrate the points in the above summary, let's examine some actual case histories of heart patients.

Case Reports

#1: J. G. R., a forty-five-year-old successful businessman, played tennis twice a week, maintained his physical fitness, and looked more thirty than fifty. During a doubles tennis match, he experienced intense pain in the pit of his stomach producing a cold sweat and causing him to stop play. He interpreted the pain as ulcer pain, the customary occupational hazard of the business world. He resumed play, suddenly collapsed, and died en route to an emergency room. At autopsy, he was found to have critical narrowing of two of his three coronary arteries. His presumed cause of death was a sudden disturbance in timing, in the rhythmicity of his heart, called **ventricular fibrillation.** Had he not misinterpreted his symptoms, his death would have been avoidable, for his coronary disease was eminently treatable.

#2: S. B. A. was a trim, active, thirty-eight-year-old schoolteacher. She had been taking birth control pills on and off for eighteen years. Her father had died of a heart attack at age forty-nine. Two of her father's brothers had died suddenly in their forties. As do many doctors and laypersons, she considered heart disease to be a man's problem. It was not of any concern to her. Her annual physical examinations consisted only of the ritual Pap smear and renewal of her birth control pills. After years of inactivity, she began jogging to shed a few pounds. She collapsed in her kitchen after one such run, and was found dead by her neighbor. Her blood fats were alarmingly high as determined by a blood sample at autopsy. She had inherited a tendency for these high blood fats (triglycerides) from her family. The levels of these blood fats were further elevated by the birth control pills. Significant in her history was that she had never experienced any ischemic pain. She never felt the warning of angina pectoris.

#3: R.W.L. was fifty-five. He had sustained a coronary occlusion three years previously. At that time, he had been hospitalized for three weeks and had been started on pills for his blood pressure, but because of problems of impotence from the blood pressure pills and because of his own wish to deny, he stopped visiting his doctor. Several months later, he began to experience an aching in the left side of his neck with mild exertion. He ignored this. A few days later he experienced the same neck discomfort at rest. He attributed the discomfort to a pulled muscle. A few days later, the neck pain returned and was followed by left arm pain. Then he felt an intense sensation of weight upon his chest, together with a profound amount of sweating and panic. There was no doubt now in his mind what he was experiencing. He has survived the heart attack but is left with about one half of the normal pumping action of his heart. Because his engine is now so inefficient, he is forced to lead an entirely sedentary existence.

#4: P. A. W. is a forty-five-year-old physician. While coaching his daughter's basketball team, he began to experience a sense of indigestion, a feeling of heartburn. With his medical knowledge, and the circumstances surrounding the exciting and trying basketball game, together with the knowledge that he had never experienced this kind of discomfort before, he immediately left the game, drove himself to an emergency room, and collapsed in the entry way of the hospital's emergency ward. He was successfully resuscitated, his heart's rhythmicity restored to normal, and subsequent therapy restored his coronary artery circulation to near normal.

Risk Factors

Who gets coronary disease? Who is most likely to develop cholesterol deposits, ischemia, angina pectoris, or myocardial infarction? In previous chapters we have talked about those factors, risk factors, most likely to produce coronary artery disease. Let us look again at the chart we examined in Chapter Seven:

Risk Factors for Coronary Artery Disease

- High blood pressure
- Obesity
- Inactivity
- Stress
- Diabetes mellitus
- Cholesterol abnormalities
- Cigarette smoking
- Dietary habits
- Family history

We have examined several of these risk factors in other chapters: cholesterol abnormalities and diabetes mellitus in Chapter Five, obesity and dietary habits in Chapter Six, the problems of the sedentary life in Chapter Seven, and cigarette smoking in Chapter Eight. Now we shall consider another important risk factor for coronary artery disease, high blood pressure.

HIGH BLOOD PRESSURE

Blood flows through the arteries of the body continuously, both when the heart squeezes and pumps (systole), as well as when the heart relaxes (diastole). The force of the blood as it flows through the arteries will be greater when the heart squeezes or pumps; blood pressure will be higher in systole than in diastole. It follows that there are two blood pressures, the **systolic** and the **diastolic** pressures. Some definitions:

If your diastolic pressure
in mmHg is: *You have:*
  less than 85   Normal blood pressure
  85-89   High normal blood pressure
  90-104   Mild high blood pressure
  105-114   Moderate high blood pressure
  greater than 115   Severe high blood pressure

If your systolic pressure
in mmHg is: *You have:*
  less than 140   Normal blood pressure
  140-159   Borderline systolic high blood
                          pressure
  greater than 160   Isolated systolic high blood
                          pressure

This defines high blood pressure. It is not a feeling of "tension," or as patients like to say "hyper-tension," nor a feeling of stress, nervousness, or anxiety. High blood pressure, or **hypertension,** is a measurement, and almost always has no symptoms associated with it. High blood pressure significantly contributes to the development of heart disease and stroke. As such, it is a leading risk factor for those two diseases. Because it has no symptoms, hypertension has been called "the silent killer." Only half of those with high blood pressure are diagnosed, and only half of those diagnosed get adequate treatment; they have either received the wrong medication or have taken the medication incorrectly.

I have a patient whose blood pressure goes up thirty or forty points when he sees me. In fact, I have many such patients. This phenomenon, that of an elevation of blood pressure when seeing a doctor, even has a name: "white-coat hypertension." Such a patient, nervous when confronted with his doctor, will also have had to contend with traffic or the weather while trying to get to his appointment. He can hardly be expected to be relaxed. To patients such as he, I suggest the purchase of a home blood pressure monitoring device.

Home Blood Pressure Monitoring

Because home blood pressure monitoring is extremely important in the therapy of a person with hypertension, you should learn the proper method of taking a blood pressure. After purchasing a blood pressure monitoring device, take it to your doctor's office to be checked for accuracy. *This is extremely important!* There is nothing worse than the false sense of security derived from an invalid blood pressure determination.

You have purchased an expensive, validated blood pressure device. You have had your doctor's office calibrate the device for accuracy. Now make sure that the size of the cuff encircles at least two thirds of your arm, having been placed as high as possible on the arm. Do not measure your blood pressure within thirty minutes of having had caffeine or nicotine. Take the measurement after five minutes of quiet rest. Measure your blood pressure at different times of day, recording the date and the time of day. If, after suitable instruction, you use the stethoscope/manometer type of blood pressure measuring device (rather than a digital electronic device), remember that the systolic pressure is that pressure at which the sound of blood spurting under the cuff appears, and the diastolic pressure is at that point when the sounds disappear, not when the sound changes in quality.

I had been following a patient with severe hypertension for several years. He was on significant doses of three different classes of medication for blood pressure and still could not be controlled. I had him come into the office at odd times of the day to have his blood pressure measured by our office nurse. With her measurements and mine, I adjusted his medications, but without success. I hospitalized him, withdrew all of his blood pressure medications, and performed laboratory testing in an attempt to diagnose some possible hormonal cause of his hypertension. There was no such hormonal cause for his blood pressure problems, as is true for about ninety percent of cases of hypertension. I put him back on medication, urged him to get his own blood pressure device to help me monitor his problem, and discharged him from the hospital.

He vanished for several months. (We call that, in the vernacular, "lost to follow-up." It happens all too frequently.) When he finally returned to the office, I asked him where he had been. His blood pressure was normal, he said. The medication was now working. He had purchased an electronic device from a local pharmacy, one that was "guaranteed," and he had checked his blood pressure everyday, even twice a day, since hospital discharge. In fact, he said, his high blood pressure was so improved, that he was able, on his own, to decrease the amount of medication he was taking.

I told him to stay in the examining room while his wife went home to get the blood pressure device. (We call that, in the vernacular, "taking a hostage.") When I compared measurements taken with his device to the measurements obtained using one of our office devices (sphygmomanometer), his true blood pressure reading was 240/150. His own device was giving him readings 30 to 40 mmHg lower than his true readings. I examined his eyes using the lighted ophthalmoscope. He had retinal hemorrhages and swelling of the optic nerve. His electrocardiogram showed the severe changes produced by the strain of this severe degree of hypertension. He was on the edge of developing a syndrome we call "malignant hypertension," a medical emergency, and life-threatening. I hospitalized him at once, started him on intravenous medicines to lower his blood pressure quickly, and kept him hospitalized until an effective anti-hypertension program could be worked out for him. His blood pressure quickly came under control with the emergency medicines. He soon left the hospital, having narrowly avoided disaster.

Treatment of Hypertension

Most commonly, the treatment of high blood pressure is lifelong. *Remember this if nothing else: Hypertension usually cannot be cured; the medicines used to control it do not produce a cure.* It is not a case of penicillin for pneumonia, for example. Drugs for hypertension are not designed to be taken for a period of time, after which they can be discarded. However, proper diet, weight reduction, exercise, and salt restriction may often control hypertension without medication, or lead to a reduction or elimination of medication in patients able to exercise such self-restraint.

It is clear now that patients with even mild hypertension (see the classifications above) should be treated. Those with high normal blood pressures should be checked yearly.

Initial therapy for high blood pressure should always include instruction for a low salt diet, weight reduction, and smoking cessation if necessary. If these measures do not result in a reduction in blood pressure, drug therapy should be started. But there is no need to rush in with two or three drugs at once, nor to take a pill containing a combination of two blood pressure medicines, especially when the high blood pressure problem is in the mild to moderate range. Time is on the side of the patient; the aim is to prevent the long-term side effects of untreated hypertension.

The decision of which medication to use should be left to your doctor. If you have followed the advice given in Chapter Two, you have found a doctor you can trust, someone who will treat your blood pressure problem correctly. Table 9-1 shows the various classes of drugs used to treat hypertension, their approximate cost per month, and their most common side effects.

TABLE 9–1   Antihypertensive Drugs

Type of Drug	Average Cost/ Month*	Common Side Effects
Diuretics ("fluid pills")		Loss of potassium, increase in
chlorothiazide (Diuril)	$ 4.50	blood sugar, rash, and other
hydrochlorothiazide (Esidrix)	3.00	allergic reactions, depression and
methyclothiazide (Enduron)	4.20	fatigue, impotence, dehydration,
polythiazide (Renese)	12.32	tendency for gout.
chlorthalidone (Hygroton)	4.50	
bumetanide (Bumex)	10.00	
furosemide (Lasix)	4.00	
Potassium-sparing diuretics		Increased potassium, rash,
spironolactone (Aldactone)	30.00	breast enlargement in males,
triamterine (Dyrenium)	32.00	menstrual problems, bone marrow disorders.
Diuretics in combination		See above.
Dyazide (hydrochlorothiazide and triamterine)	6.30	
Maxzide (hydrochlorothiazide and triamterine)	11.15	
Aldactazide (hydrochlorothiazide and spironolactone)	31.50	
Moduretic (hydrochlorothiazide and amiloride)	9.35	
Beta-blockers		Fatigue, slow pulse, depression,
acebutolol (Sectral)	32.75	asthma-like condition, night-
metoprolol (Lopressor)	15.20	mares, whitening of the fingers.
nadolol (Corgard)	14.40	
pindolol (Visken)	34.50	
atenolol (Tenormin)	15.30	
labetolol (Trandate, Normodyne)	23.75	
timolol (Blocadren)	26.45	
propranolol (Inderal)	21.30	
Blood vessel dilators		Dizziness with changes in
guanethidine (Ismelin)	19.50	posture, retention of fluid, head-
prazosin (Minipress)	21.00	ache, drowsiness, depression.
reserpine (Serpasil)		
Drugs acting within the brain		Headache, insomnia, depression.
clonidine (Catapres)	10.80	
guanabenz (Wytensin)	35.72	
methyldopa (Aldomet)	14.12	

TABLE 9–1   continued

Type of Drug	Average Cost/ Month*	Common Side Effects
Artery dilators		
hydralazine (Apresoline)	8.72	Rapid pulse, aggravation of angina pectoris, headache, dizziness, rash.
minoxidil (Loniten)	20.00	Rapid pulse, aggravation of angina, fluid retention, hair growth on face and body, coarsening of facial features.
Blood pressure-hormone inhibitors *(angiotensin-converting enzyme inhibitors)*		Loss of taste and appetite, rash,
captopril (Capoten)	32.40	cough, severe kidney problems,
enalopril (Vasotec)	17.09	jaundice.
lisinopril (Zestril)	18.62	
Calcium antagonists		Disturbances of heart rhythm,
diltiazem (Cardizem)	43.19	headache, fatigue, fluid build
nifedipine (Procardia)	28.25	up, rash.
verapamil (Calan, Isoptin)	19.25	

Note: Generic drugs are not capitalized.

*Prices are for average doses, and for generic drugs where available, as of December, 1988.

Cautionary Notes About High Blood Pressure

Before we leave our discussion of hypertension, we should clear up a few misconceptions. Meditation, or "the relaxation response," although highly publicized, has been studied carefully as a possible means of controlling hypertension, and has been found wanting. The results of these medical studies have shown that this form of therapy has no affect on established high blood pressure. It does *not* eliminate the need for drug therapy. Remember also that there is a vast difference between treatment and cure. Insulin treats diabetes mellitus; it does not cure diabetes. Similarly, drugs for hypertension treat or control the disease; they do not cure it. Treatment for hypertension is lifelong. Another point: *treatment must be individualized.* What works for one person will not work for another. One patient may experience side effects with a drug well tolerated by another patient. As the list above makes clear, there are a whole variety of drugs for high blood pressure; almost always a drug treatment regimen can be found for every individual patient. *Understand the medication you are taking, its side effects, the proper dose and dosing intervals, and communicate to your doctor any and all problems you are having with the medication.* This includes, most especially, those men who experience impotence from some of these medications.

CORONARY ARTERY DISEASE

The most typical thing about angina pectoris, heart pain, is that it is atypical. One patient experiences the "classical" symptom of a heavy weight in the center of the chest associated with exercise or emotion. Another patient feels only a sense of heartburn or indigestion in the pit of the stomach while another may feel a burning or aching in the side of the neck, either side. Some patients may feel only left arm discomfort, and one patient, shortly before a heart attack, complained to me of pain *only* in the palm of his left hand.

I remember that patient well. I was making rounds in the hospital one Sunday morning when I came upon the patient, an elderly Finn of few words. He was standing in the hall, leaning against a railing. His forehead was beaded with sweat. I asked him what was the matter.

"Pain," he said.

I asked him where he had pain. He pointed to the palm of his left hand. I asked him if he had pain anywhere else. He shook his head no. I asked him how bad the pain was.

"Bad," he said.

Something about him made me very nervous. I asked the nurses to get an electrocardiogram on him immediately. The electrocardiogram showed changes diagnostic of an impending heart attack. We rushed him to the intensive care unit. He was given medicines (discussed below) which aborted his heart attack and spared him extensive damage to his heart muscle.

Diagnosis of Coronary Artery Disease

Diagnosis is difficult business! How can one anticipate coronary disease? *Keep the risk factors in mind.* If you are at increased risk for developing problems of coronary artery disease, if your family history is against you, you have high blood pressure, or if you are overweight and sedentary, be very attentive to any kind of discomfort, especially that associated with exercise or emotion. As in many areas of medicine, this is where having a doctor you trust and can communicate with is so vitally important. If a patient calls me and says, "Doc, for the past few weeks I have been having this problem. Everytime I climb a flight of stairs at work, I get this funny feeling in my chest." A complaint like that deserves an immediate evaluation for coronary artery disease!

The complaints vary, but the theme is the same:

"Everytime my wife and I have an argument, I get indigestion during the argument."

"This year, for the first time, when I begin shoveling snow, I get short of breath." (From a forty-five-year-old man)

"I'm active . . . but it's funny . . . if I walk outside, especially if I walk quickly, and especially if it's cold out, I get this funny burning in my left shoulder."

"I can do most anything. But if I eat a heavy meal and then I try to exercise, I get an ache, not really a pain, just an ache, in my chest."

For the alert physician, and for the informed lay person, the diagnosis here is easy: Discomfort in the chest, neck, jaw, or arms, when associated with exercise or emotion, often signals *critical* coronary artery disease.

But what about the patient, S. B. A., the young woman who had no symptoms at all and collapsed in her kitchen? These cases are more difficult. A thorough, complete periodic physical examination is of paramount importance, as is corresponding periodic laboratory testing. Remember the advice in Chapter Seven: Any sedentary adult contemplating an exercise program should consider exercise testing by a physician first.

Treatment of Coronary Artery Disease

The treatment of plugged coronary arteries has undergone a revolution in the past twenty years. Twenty years ago a patient was "allowed" to have his or her heart attack, while we physicians stood by treating the pain and trying to ward off any disturbances in rhythm. It was the standard then to keep patients in the hospital for two or three weeks, treat them as invalids, and not permit them even to sit up by themselves.

Then came the era of surgical treatment of coronary disease. With the development of the technique of **bypass grafting,** restoration of blood flow with relief of angina pectoris and prevention of heart attacks became possible. In this technique, still commonly performed, a piece of vein from a leg vessel is sewn onto the blocked coronary artery, both before and after the blockage, to provide a detour passage around which blood can flow. And because the coronary arteries lie on the surface of the heart, they are readily accessible to the surgeon's skill.

Balloon Angioplasty

More recently, less drastic therapy has been developed. This technique, called PCTA (percutaneous transluminal angioplasty), involves the use of a small plastic catheter inserted in a leg artery and then passed upward to the area of the heart. Using X-ray for guidance, the plastic catheter is selectively passed into the diseased coronary artery and positioned so that its tip lies within the area of critical blockage. In this position, a small balloon is blown up at the tip of the catheter, and the blockage is "cracked" open. Instead of an "open-chest" heart operation and several days to weeks in the hospital, a patient can be treated with PCTA and leave the hospital the next day.

PCTA is not for everyone; in many cases there are multiple areas of blockage which require bypass grafting by a surgeon. Or the blockage can be in an area of an artery very difficult to reach with a catheter. Sometimes, patients treated with PCTA may quickly 're-plug' the artery and, usually within six months of the PCTA, begin again to experience angina. Close follow-up by physicians is mandatory for these patients.

Dissolving Blood Clots

A fifty-five-year-old patient came to the emergency room within thirty minutes of developing severe, unremitting chest pain. He characterized his pain as "the most severe pain I had ever experienced, compounded by a sense of dread, of impending doom." His electrocardiogram showed changes indicating the beginnning of a very large myocardial infarction, or heart attack. The patient was immediately given an injection of a medication by vein, followed thereafter by a continuous infusion of a second medication to prevent his blood from clotting. Within the hour his pain was gone. He felt "normal." His electrocardiogram had returned to normal.

Because his pain recurred, and because of his electrocardiographic changes at the time of his pain, he was immediately transferred to a large referral hospital where his coronary arteries were X-rayed on an emergency basis. He was found to have an almost total blockage of the left main coronary artery — a blockage anatomists once callously referred to as "the widowmaker." (See Figure 9-2. The three main coronary arteries are derived from only two routes or trunks. The artery labeled "3" in Figure 9-2, the right coronary artery, arises from one trunk and the two arteries labeled "4" and "5," the left anterior descending artery and the left circumflex artery, branch from a single trunk, the left main coronary artery. Now you can begin to appreciate the importance of the left main coronary artery.)

This patient's left main coronary artery disease was treated with PCTA (the balloon surgery). He was discharged from the hospital in a few days without having suffered any permanent damage to his heart muscle.

But the story does not end there; he appreciated how close he had come. Through dieting and dietary restriction he has lost fifty-five pounds and has decreased his serum cholesterol by one hundred points.

This patient's heart muscle, indeed his very life, was saved by the prompt administration of a clot-dissolving substance. The use of this substance, called **thrombolytic therapy,** has revolutionized further the treatment of heart attacks; prompt administration of the drug early in the course of a heart attack can limit dramatically the amount of heart muscle damaged. It may prevent damage entirely. The drug is called tissue plasminogen activator, or TPA, and the results have been fantastic. If we can treat a patient with the drug within a half an hour of the onset of symptoms, we are very likely to prevent heart muscle damage entirely. If TPA is given within an hour of onset of symptoms, between fifty and eighty percent of the threatened heart muscle can still be saved. If the patient waits for longer than four hours before coming to the hospital, the results are far less spectacular. After six hours, we do not administer the drug.

The most exciting aspect of this thrombolytic therapy with TPA is that the drug can be given in any hospital! The drug is administered through a peripheral vein. Protocol requires only that a trained physician be in attendance and that certain contraindications — recent surgery, prior history of brain hemorrhage, occult gastrointestinal bleeding, for example — are not present. Consider the implications of this discovery! An effective therapy for a lethal disease has been developed and refined to the point where it is on the front lines, where the patients are. This is not therapy for the ivory tower, but therapy for the masses, *which is what medicine and doctoring are all about.*

Medical Therapy for Angina Pectoris

TPA does not dissolve cholesterol deposits. Not all patients are candidates for bypass surgery. What about the elderly person with mild angina pectoris who wants to remain active but is prevented from doing so by chest pain? What about our young patient in his forties (discussed in Chapter Seven) with severe, diffuse coronary artery disease that could not be bypassed surgically? What of the patient with severe coronary artery disease whose other medical problems prevent major surgery?

There is still much that can be done. Medications of the class **beta-blockers** decrease the work of the heart, the force of contraction of the muscle-pump. When demand upon the heart is increased, for example at tax time or with the first snowfall, the heart treated with beta-blockers does not respond as forcefully to this demand. Ischemia and angina pectoris are prevented. The more common beta-blockers, their side effects and cost, are listed above in the discussion on treatment of hypertension.

A new class of drugs, the **calcium channel blockers,** also listed in the section on treatment of hypertension, have added a new dimension to the medical therapy of angina pectoris. By dilating, or widening, the coronary arteries and therefore increasing blood flow, and by reducing the load upon the heart in certain other ways, these agents effectively treat angina pectoris.

Over one hundred years ago severe angina pectoris was treated by eminent physicians with bloodletting. It was observed that when a patient was "bled," (a common treatment for most diseases those days) the patient's angina pectoris was temporarily relieved. It was postulated, correctly, that this was because of a lowering of blood pressure. Certain nitrogen compounds, nitrates and nitrites, and most notably nitroglycerin, were found to do the same thing: They profoundly lowered the patient's blood pressure and relieved angina pectoris for varying periods of time. Today nitrates and nitrites are still commonly (and correctly) used as an adjunct in the treatment of angina pectoris.

One hundred and fifty years ago physicians, when confronted with a heart patient, applied leeches, bled the patient, offered a few leaves of the digitalis plant for thorough chewing, and prayed. How far medicine has come! Exciting therapy has transformed the treatment of coronary artery disease. For the patient, the message is clear: Pay attention to risk factors. Be sensitive to any symptoms suggestive of coronary disease. Be aware of the miracle of prompt, early therapy. *It is a matter of life and death.*

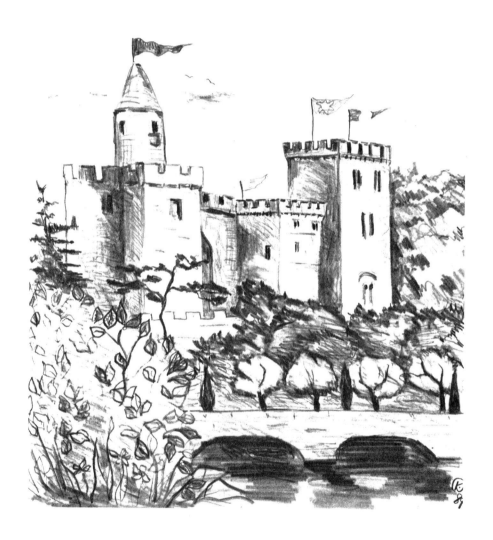

10

Cancer

"An evil disease, say they, cleaveth fast unto him; and now that he lieth he shall rise up no more."

Psalm 41:8

Imagine you live in a grand palace. This palace has an
infinite number of rooms with all the modern con-
veniences. There is central heating, of course, and
central air-conditioning for those intolerably humid
summer days. Every room has a fireplace. There is
central vacuuming and a vast central kitchen connected
to dumbwaiters, elevators, and message tubes to carry
menus, food, and complaints about the soup to every
room and every wing of the palace. Because you have so
much room, your children are allowed pets of any and
every description: dogs, cats, a clutch of hamsters,
assorted gerbils, parakeets, canaries — even a snake or
two.

Your palace is the picture of tranquility — order
and discipline are everywhere. Security is ensured
within by an internal alarm system, and, outside, by
the customary palace guards. Every living thing in the
palace has its rightful place. The palace itself, filled
with life, purrs along in predictable fashion. Your
palace itself becomes some grand organism.

Now imagine that something goes haywire with
the plant life in your palace. All the vegetation, once
shelved, potted, and restrained, grows without reason,
unchecked. Philodendrons possess the conservatory.
Schefflera command the library, insinuating tendrils
between and among the volumes, carpeting the floor
with dull green foliage, clinging to fixtures in jungle-like
fashion. Their roots clog the message tubes. The ivy
clogs the dumbwaiters. Every hall is choked with
geraniums. The guest bedrooms become filled with
pachysandra.

Your palace and every living thing in it are
threatened by this wanton proliferation. What do you
do?

The solution is simple. You find an effective
herbicide with minimal toxicity to animal life, use the
herbicide in moderation, and relentlessly spray until
the palace is yours again. Because plants are essentially
different from animals, you can exploit that difference
by selecting an herbicide which preferentially kills the

unwanted vegetation, while leaving your family and pets unscathed.

Imagine now that the grand palace is the human body, that the family, pets, dumbwaiters, and appliances comprise every form of life within the human body. This invasion of vegetation can then be likened to a bacterial infection. Certain herbicides, called **antibiotics,** exploit the difference between bacteria (plants) and animal tissue (that is, the family and pets residing within the palace).

This is the situation we will deal with in Chapter 12, "Common Infections." It is mentioned here so you will be able to distinguish it from the problem we face with cancer, wherein it is the palace's *animal* life, rather than its plant life, which is attempting the takeover.

Consider this frightening scenario: Your palace, warm against the November night, amber-lit in the dusk, rests in seeming security. The palace guards stand alert, ready to deny admission to any foreign thing. The internal security system, ever vigilant, keeps a twenty-four hour watch against any unlikely invasion from within. Any cat, dog, or gerbil that is not your own will be recognized immediately by your security system and dealt with severely. But what happens is altogether unprepared for. One gerbil reproduces, reproduces again, and again, and so on, in geometric fashion, doubling its numbers again and again: two, then four, then eight, sixteen . . .

In no time the palace is overrun by gerbils. Though the palace and its intricate workings are threatened by this unbridled reproduction of a single pet, your security system is not sensitive enough to tell the difference between the gerbil and its progeny. Moreover, since gerbils are not plants, they are similar to other animal inhabitants of the palace. You may set out "gerbil-poison" and kill the gerbils, but you will certainly poison the other pets as well. You may spray generous amounts of rodenticide but you will certainly kill your hamsters and probably your family in the process.

This is the metaphor for cancer. The offending

cancer cell (gerbil) looks almost identical to the permanent residents of your palace (the human body). The difference between the unwanted gerbils and the original pet is very slight indeed and can only be recognized by experts. Within the palace, in fact, the difference between gerbils and other living things (other pets and your family, for example) is negligible as well. One would like to find a "gerbil-cide" which will kill only gerbils. Ideally, one would like a "gerbil-cide" which kills only the unwanted offspring of the one gerbil that began this senseless replication, leaving alone all of the other pet gerbils which are still wanted, and are, in the metaphorical sense, necessary for the completeness of the palace.

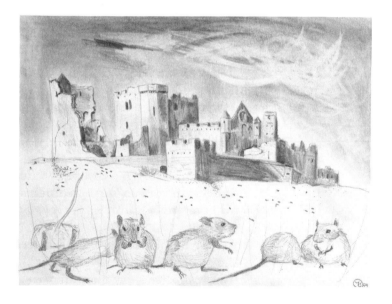

THE NATURE OF CANCER

That is the picture of cancer as a process. Cancer is neither an Evil Thing nor a moral judgment. Cancer does not kill merely by being there. *Given time for enough reproduction,* the vast numbers of cancer cells overrun the body, interfere with its function, and cause the death of the organism through interference with breathing, waste elimination, or any other body function. In our metaphor, the horde of gerbils overruns the kitchen, consumes all the food, and chokes the dumbwaiters, elevators, ventilation system, and message tubes.

How do you avoid a palace full of unwanted gerbils? In Chapter Four we discussed carcinogens, the cancer-causing agents, as well as the hazards of radiation. An ounce of prevention is worth a pound of cure. There are surveillance systems (medical testing devices) and individuals (doctors) sophisticated enough to tell when the gerbils are *beginning* to get out of hand, and in some instances even *anticipate* when the gerbils might do so. Certain common sense advice, apparent to any layperson, may also prevent invasion by gerbils: Keep the cages locked, prevent fraternization among gerbils, don't give them the run of the house with gerbil food sprinkled everywhere, and keep a periodic check on what the gerbils are up to.

This palace-metaphor is very useful. We shall return to it from time to time when considering specific common cancers in this chapter and certain infections in Chapter Twelve. But now, as we turn to specific common malignancies, remember these few points about the palace-metaphor:

- One, solitary cage full of unwanted gerbils does not mean that the palace is lost.
- A given palace (human being) may have a tendency towards unwanted reproduction of a certain part of its whole (an inherited tendency towards certain cancers). What is the history of your house?
- Unchecked reproduction of certain elements of the palace is far worse than for other such elements. For example, unchecked reproduction of the palace guards and/or the security system is far worse than a bit of scaly lichen on the roof of the south tower.
- Effective surveillance systems exist to screen for things amiss within the palace. The systems are expensive, a nuisance, and can be used only

periodically. Who wants to live in a palace continually patrolled by a police force or an army of
exterminators?

- Feed your palace guards well, give them adequate
rest and vacation, and freedom from stress and
strain, and they will serve you well. Beat the
guards down with twenty-four hours of alarm,
with continual attack and insult upon the palace,
and the guards will wear down as they must.

- As the palace grows old, the bells, whistles, wires
and diodes of its alarm system will wear down, in
some cases short out, and become less efficient at
protecting the whole.

BREAST CANCER

Let's get a sense of proportion about this disease! Since
the AIDS pandemic was initially recognized in 1981, an
estimated 250,000 cases of AIDS have occurred *worldwide.* Since 1981 alone, 280,000 women have died of
breast cancer *just in America.* Yet I would submit that
the average high school girl's perception of risk for
contracting AIDS is much higher than her perception
of risk of breast cancer. Yet, breast cancer, in its earliest
stages, is almost always curable, while AIDS, once it
has developed, reaches a fatality rate of one hundred
percent.

Who Is at Risk?

Just as there are certain lifestyles and conditions —risk
factors — for the development of heart disease, so there
are certain conditions predisposing a woman to breast
cancer. What are the risk factors?

- Women whose mothers and/or sisters have had
breast cancers have a three to four-fold increase in
the risk of developing breast cancer themselves.

- A woman who has had breast cancer before has an
equal increase in risk as well.

- Women who have never been pregnant, get pregnant after age thirty for the first time, have very
early onset of menstruation, or very late menopause
are at increased risk.

- If a woman's mother was premenopausal when her breast cancer developed, or if a woman has both a mother and a sister with breast cancer, that woman's risk is magnified.

What conditions and/or lifestyles are *not* associated with an increased risk for breast cancer? Women who have breasts containing scars and cysts, so-called **fibrocystic** disease of the breast, do not have a higher risk of breast cancer. Women who consume alcohol or take birth control pills likewise do *not* have a higher risk of breast cancer. Whether diet, especially a diet high in the consumption of animal fats, plays a role in the development of breast cancer is debatable; there are medical studies suggesting that obesity itself is a risk factor for breast cancer and other studies suggesting that high animal-fat consumption may increase the risk of developing breast cancer. Breast-feeding does not lower the risk of breast cancer in a woman. Whether exercise lowers risk is also debatable, but one study has shown a 35 percent lower breast cancer rate among former women athletes.

Risk Factors for Breast Cancer

- Family history (especially mother or sister)
- Prior breast cancer
- No pregnancies
- First pregnancy age greater than thirty
- Early onset of menstruation
- Late menopause
- Obesity (?)
- Lack of exercise (?)
- A diet high in animal fat (?)

Conditions That Do Not Place You at Risk for Breast Cancer

- Alcohol consumption
- Birth control pills
- Use of oral estrogens after menopause
- Failure to breast-feed
- Fibrocystic disease of the breast

Catch Those Gerbils Early!

The more the gerbils are given the run of the house, the less likely it becomes that you can restore your palace to its former healthy state. Identify the frenzied reproduction of your pet gerbils in their early stages — that is, diagnose a breast cancer growing **in situ** (only at its place of origin) — and you can call the exterminator (the surgeon) who will remove the problem for you and have done with it. Catching it *early* is key. But how does one make an early diagnosis of breast cancer?

Breast Cancer Screening

Early detection of breast cancer — and high rate of cure — depend upon four screening maneuvers:

- Periodic mammography
- Breast self-examination
- Periodic breast examination by a physician
- Biopsy of all suspicious breast masses

Some Case Histories

Patient A is a forty-one-year-old mother of two. She has no family history of breast cancer, performs monthly breast self-examination, and has a yearly breast examination by her physician. She is of normal weight, has no fibrocystic disease of her breasts (therefore her breasts are easy to examine), and is advised to get breast X-rays, **mammograms,** every other year. She is performing adequate and highly reliable screening for breast cancer.

Patient B, a thirty-one-year-old registered nurse, performs monthly breast self-examination, gets a yearly examination by her physician, and yearly mammograms. Her sister died at age twenty-nine of breast cancer. She *too* is performing adequate, highly reliable screening for breast cancer.

Patient C is a thirty-three-year-old mother of two. Her mother developed breast cancer at age fifty-three, after menopause. The patient, because of her mother's disease, began to do monthly breast self-examination in her twenties. Because she detected a lump which appeared new to her and had not been there before, she brought it to her physician's attention. (Most breast cancers are found by patients, not doctors.) Because the patient was confident in her own breast self-examination and reliable in her assessment that this was a new lump, the suspicious lump was biopsied. It was a very early breast cancer, a cancer in situ. She was treated successfully with surgical removal of the lump and with breast radiation therapy after surgery.

Patient D, now forty-four years old, is dying of breast cancer. The cancer has spread to her bones, eroding the bone, causing severe pain, as well as problems with her calcium metabolism. The cancer has spread to her liver, replacing normal liver tissue and interfering with her body's liver function. And, if she survives long enough, her breast cancer may spread to her brain. Yet she had detected her own breast cancer at a very early, in situ, stage. What had gone wrong?

Eleven years before, in the course of performing monthly breast self-examination, Patient D had detected a suspicious lump. Although she had no family history of breast cancer and no other risk factors for the development of breast cancer, she was certain that this lump was new. Over the course of a few months, she felt that the lump was enlarging, however slowly. She brought the lump to the attention of her physician, who immediately ordered mammograms. The mammograms were negative, that is, they did not show evidence of change suggestive of breast cancer. Nevertheless, because of the patient's reliability, because of her assessment that the lump was enlarging, her physician referred her to a surgeon for biopsy of the breast lump.

It was here that several things went wrong. The surgeon decided "to wait and see." The *primary physician* had turned his patient over to the surgeon, trusting that the lump would be biopsied. The primary physician did not have a check and balance system in place to be sure that immediate biopsy would be performed. The patient herself had assumed that she had been "turned over" to the surgeon, and that the surgeon knew best. The patient therefore never communicated back to her primary physician that biopsy would be delayed.

The biopsy *was* delayed, for eight months. When

the lump was finally biopsied and found cancerous, its cancer cells had already spread to the patient's lymph glands adjacent to her breast. First with surgery, and then with repeated courses of chemotherapy, the patient has been fighting a losing battle against her disease.

It is impossible to say which of the four screening maneuvers is most important. Monthly self-examination, yearly examination by a physician, routine periodic mammograms, biopsy of all suspicious lesions — *all* are extremely important. But of these screening tests, periodic mammography, although extremely sensitive in detecting cancers and crucial in the diagnosis of breast cancer, is shockingly underplayed. Mammography, (breast X-rays), can pick up a breast cancer as early as two years before it can be felt. Many groups are culpable for this under-use of mammography. Some doctors remain unconvinced of its usefulness, or "forget" to order them. Patients worry that the radiation involved in breast X-rays is itself harmful or cancer causing — *not true!* The test itself is expensive, and patients are reluctant to pay for it — as are insurance carriers who balk at paying for "routine" testing. In fact, most insurance carriers have assumed the ridiculous posture of refusing to pay for any cancer screening, while footing the enormous bills resulting from care of the dying cancer patient. What mammography needs is the same media blitz that has occurred for cholesterol screening. Women need to besiege their doctors with requests for mammography. In fact, my advice is even stronger: if you are over forty and your doctor does not advise mammography, turn to Chapter Two in this book and begin the search for a new doctor.

Treatment of Breast Cancer

It used to be that finding a cancer, no matter how early, meant losing your breast. That was enough to discourage any woman from breast cancer surveillance. Today the choices of treatment for early breast cancer are many. A woman may have a simple mastectomy, that is, the breast containing the cancer is removed together with sampling of the lymph glands in the area to see whether and how far the disease has spread. A woman may alternatively consider removal of just the lump, followed by radiation of the entire breast, as did our young woman, Patient C. In some cases, removal of the lump without any further therapy is sufficient. Here is the advice I give any woman coming to me who is found to have breast cancer:

Any woman with breast cancer should obtain multiple opinions with regard to treatments, from cancer specialists (oncologists) and surgeons, as well as from her primary doctor.

Even when surgery must be drastic, the outcome today need not be mutilating. *A story* . . . .

A young woman came to her internist with her complaint of having felt a new breast lump. Although she was extremely thin, and her breasts small, she had a considerable amount of scarring and cyst formation (fibrocystic breasts) which made her breasts very difficult to examine. Nevertheless, she was adamant that the lump she had found was new. Her mammograms showed only the fibrocystic disease. They were not diagnostic of any early breast cancer. Nevertheless, the suspicious lump was removed. It was a very early breast cancer, *in situ,* of a peculiar and unusual cell type. In brief, given this particular kind of breast cancer, the woman was at increased risk of developing similar cancers elsewhere in either breast. Her surgeon recommended close surveillance, that is, periodic mammography, periodic physician-breast examination, and monthly breast examinations by the patient herself. But would that be sufficient? The mammograms had not shown anything anyway, even though biopsy had proven an early cancer. And the patient had such extensive fibrocystic changes that the physician could not tell one lump from another, even though the patient had found the lump. Could the patient be relied upon to pick up another early cancer? Would another early cancer arise in an area of her breast easily accessible to her palpating fingers? Several oncologists were consulted, both by the patient and by the patient's primary physician. Ultimately, after all of these consultations, the patient and her husband chose bilateral mastectomies, that is, removal of both breasts. Her doctor agreed with this decision.

The patient was referred to a large medical center where *both* mastectomies could be done in the same surgical procedure, together with breast reconstruction by a plastic surgeon during that same surgery. When the patient awoke from her surgery she had "new" breasts rather than none at all.

> *But the story goes further, and there is a moral: Her husband was with her every step of the way. Through all of the consultations and choices to be made, he supported her decisions and, most importantly, was thrilled for her with the results of her plastic surgery. It is a rare woman indeed who does not think, when a breast cancer is diagnosed, "What will my husband think?"*

COLON CANCER

Even in the nether regions of the palace, dark and malignant things may grow. Cancer of the colon and rectum is an extremely common malignancy. Who gets this disease? What are its risk factors?

Habit of diet seems to be extremely important in colon/rectum cancer. High fiber diets seem to protect those societies whose diets are predisposed to roughage. One theory is that fiber in the diet increases the movement of waste through the bowels, thereby decreasing the length of time during which the colon may be exposed to cancer-causing agents in the diet (carcinogens). A diet low in animal fats also seems to protect against the development of colon cancer. In geographic areas where meat is consumed in high quantities, there is an increased incidence of colon tumors. There is research evidence as well that dietary calcium may inactivate certain carcinogens in the diet and protect against the development of cancer of the bowel. Remember, though, that these theories of diet are *theories;* there is no conclusive proof of any *single* diet or dietary habit which either causes or protects one against colon cancer.

Other Risk Factors

Heredity is an extremely important risk factor for colorectal cancer. One-quarter of patients with colorectal cancer have a family history of that cancer. Clearly then, a patient whose family has a history of cancer of the rectum or colon is at increased risk of developing the disease himself. The man whose family history includes the occurrence of colorectal cancer is at similar risk as the woman with a strong family history of breast cancer. For both patients, increased surveillance is mandatory.

There are two other high risk conditions worthy of consideration. Certain forms of **colitis,** of longstanding duration, predispose to the development of cancers. These inflammatory conditions are not the common garden-variety spasms of the colon from which we all suffer, spasms sporadic and self-limited in nature. Inflammatory bowel diseases are in themselves serious conditions, uncommon, and debilitating. Those suffering with such a disease for several years are at increased risk for colon cancer.

Another high risk condition is the existence of **polyps.** Most cancers of the rectum and colon develop from benign noncancerous polyps. In the course of screening procedures and routine examinations, if a person is found to be prone to the development of polyps, that person is at increased risk and requires increased surveillance for the appearance of colon cancer.

Conditions *Increasing* the Risk of Colorectal Cancer

- Family history
- Prior colon malignancy
- Existence of polyps
- A diet high in animal fats
- A diet low in fiber
- A low dietary calcium (?)
- A diet low in cabbage, Brussels sprouts, broccoli (?)
- Long-standing inflammatory bowel disease

How does colorectal cancer kill? Remember our palace metaphor. A small nest of gerbils somewhere deep in the basement begins to proliferate furiously. Unchecked, the gerbils invade the message tubes of the palace and run rampant throughout its system. They invade the palace's decontamination system (the liver), its internal defense system (the lymph glands), its ventilation system (the lungs), and its very structural bulwarks (the bones). Once it has spread so widely throughout the palace, colorectal cancer is, in our present state of knowledge, untreatable. Confined to the basement, and still localized, the nest of cancer is relatively easy to detect and available to the surgeon's knife for cure.

Screening for Colorectal Cancer

The asymptomatic individual who has no high risk conditions (no family history, no history of polyps, no history of inflammatory bowel disease) should submit to the following cancer screening procedures to guard against cancer of the rectum and colon:

- Flexible fiberoptic sigmoidoscopy
- Stool guaiac slide testing (test for occult blood)
- Examination of the rectum by a physician

What are these procedures and how often should they be performed? The **sigmoidoscopy** is an office procedure performed by an *experienced* physician with a lighted flexible tube inserted into the rectum. With this tube, the physician examines some 60 centimeters of rectum and lower colon, the most common sites of origin of colorectal cancers. After age fifty, everyone should have two such negative examinations one year apart and then periodic sigmoidoscopies every three to five years after that. There are some key points to remember about this examination:

- Examination with a shorter, rigid tube of some 25 centimeters is *not* sufficient.
- Examination by an experienced physician who performs these procedures *daily* is preferable. (Early cancers are not always obvious.)
- Those at high risk (polyps, family history) should

submit to the examination more frequently, as advised by their physician.

- Those with strong family histories, especially family history of multiple colon polyps, should begin such examinations at a much earlier age, as advised by their physician.

Bowel cancers may bleed, often very early in their development. The blood in the feces may be fairly obvious, rendering the stool a dark maroon color, or, if the blood is digested, jet-black. More often, however, the presence of blood in the stool is not apparent. A chemical test for the presence of small amounts of blood, the **stool guaiac slide test,** is easily performed. How often this should be done is debatable, and varies from physician to physician. We ask our patients over age fifty to send in such a test every two to three months. The test is simply performed; the slides or cards are obtained from your physician's office. A small amount of feces is smeared on the card, enclosed, and mailed to the physician. Chemical is added to the card which will, in the presence of blood, produce an intense blue color. When a test is positive, we ask the patient to repeat three to six more tests on a daily basis, avoiding any irritants to the bowel such as aspirin or iron therapy, as well as any meat products that may contain animal blood and will give a falsely positive test. It is important to remember when performing the test to avoid taking vitamin C in tablet form, which may cause the test to be falsely negative. Remember, too, that this is *not* a highly reliable form of screening and is to be done *in addition to* sigmoidoscopy and rectal examination by your physician. Probably as many as *fifty percent* of patients with a known bowel cancer will fail to show traces of blood in the stool with this test. In addition, polyps rarely bleed and, as mentioned above, may be precancerous. They can only be detected with the flexible fiberoptic sigmoidoscopy.

Finally, everyone over age forty should have an annual rectal examination by his or her physician. This rectal examination is not only useful for screening for colorectal cancer, but is also the best screening test for prostate cancer in men and should be part of the pelvic examination for women anyway. As a part of this rectal examination, the physician himself will perform a stool guaiac slide test on the spot.

Early Symptoms of Colon Cancer

Bowel cancers become increasingly common with advancing age. After age fifty, a *change in bowel habits* may be an early symptom of colorectal cancer. The appearance of abdominal cramping, constipation, or diarrhea where none existed before should always be a warning signal to patient and doctor, especially in patients over fifty. Tumors may bleed, as discussed above, and produce an anemia with symptoms of lassitude and easy fatiguing. And, finally, obvious rectal bleeding should *always* be considered a warning of cancer until proven otherwise. Many are the patients and physicians who falsely attribute this bleeding to hemorrhoids. The best advice is this: *Always assume the worst and work hard to prove it false.*

I had a patient, a young man of forty-eight, who observed bright red rectal bleeding in himself. As he would later tell me, he immediately knew he had cancer. At the time he noted the bleeding, he made a common erroneous assumption: that the presence of a cancer always means certain death. Since he believed this to be true, his highest priority was to get his affairs in order. He finished building and insulating his house for his family, a job which took some eight months. By the time he came to me to have his problem taken care of, his rectal cancer had spread to his lymph glands and to his liver. He died a few months later. Had his first priority been himself, his cancer in all likelihood would have been curable at the time of the bleeding, curable through surgical excision. And his family would still have him.

Since the time of Hippocrates and Galen, early diagnosis of cancer has been stressed to patient and physician. When physicians stress annual checkups, they are talking in part about cancer screening. When patients come to physicians "to catch it early," they are thinking about cancer. *As in so many diseases, the best treatment for cancer is early detection.*

LUNG CANCER

Imagine the immense task asked of the ventilation system of your palace. This system warms, filters, conditions, and processes the external atmosphere to provide clean air for your family and pets to breathe. And there's the rub! The ventilation system is asked to process polluted gas, an atmosphere containing tobacco smoke, radon, petrochemicals, asbestos, and other cancer-causing chemicals. Not only does this harsh external atmosphere grind and tear at the ventilation system, producing chronic debilitating diseases (such as emphysema and chronic bronchitis), but these chemicals, carcinogens, also cause rapid uncontrolled reproduction of particularly nasty gerbils. These malignant nests of rodents, lung cancers, tend to spread to other parts of the palace very early, almost before their senseless replication is noticed at the original site. This means that usually by the time a gerbil problem is identified in the ventilatory system, it is almost always too late to do anything about it. There simply exists no reliable screening and detection program for the diagnosis of lung cancer. Pap smears are extremely helpful in diagnosing an early cancer of the cervix. Rectal exams are the key to the diagnosis of cancer of the prostate. Mammography and flexible fiberoptic sigmoidoscopy are extremely helpful tools in finding breast and colon cancers before they have spread. But there is as yet no such tool for lung cancer. Several large research studies have shown that screening chest X-rays do not improve survival of lung cancer in *any* large group studied.

Who is at high risk? We have examined this in Chapters Four and Eight, the chapters on preventive medicine and tobacco abuse. However, here is a review.

High Risk Conditions for Lung Cancer

- Smoking cigarettes
- Working with asbestos
- Smoking cigarettes
- Working in a mine
- Smoking cigarettes
- Exposure to radon gas
- Smoking marijuana
- Smoking cigarettes

Rarely are people cured of lung cancer. Those fortunate enough to survive generally fall into two groups: those whose cancers are found by chance on a routine chest X-ray and surgically removed before spreading has occurred and those who have an uncommon type of lung cancer, oat cell cancer of the lung, which has a better chance of responding to chemotherapy than the usual tobacco-caused lung cancer. *Nevertheless, the mortality for all kinds of lung cancer, oat cell and otherwise, is very high.*

Prevention of Lung Cancer

Prevention of lung cancer is simple. You already know the answer. Without tobacco, lung cancer would be an extremely uncommon disease. Since 1985, because of cigarette smoking, lung cancer has caused more deaths in both men and women than any other type of cancer in the United States. Consider the implications of this! What other product that we buy has a label warning us that it causes cancer? When we worry about the costs of health care, when we busy ourselves with lawsuits against those who injure us, those who deprive us of our happiness and our loved ones, what do we make of tobacco subsidies? Is there any justification for higher insurance premiums for cigarette smokers? Should cigarette smokers be insured at all? Forewarned, should cigarette smokers be permitted to sue tobacco companies? Or sue doctors? Or hospitals? Why is our perceived risk for cigarette smoking so small compared to, let's say, nuclear power? Could it have anything to do with television, theater, the media, and the tobacco companies themselves?

CANCER OF THE PROSTATE

Prostate cancer is quite common. It is a condition both of male-ness and of advancing age. It does not occur in eunuchs and is rare before age sixty. Differences in the occurrence of prostate cancer among black men in the United States (high) and Japanese men in the Orient (very low) suggest some possible environmental cause. But neither an environmental cause nor any definite risk factors for prostate cancer have been identified. Prostate cancer is one of the major cancers *not* associated with cigarette smoking. Nor have radiation exposure and diet been implicated in the appearance of prostate cancer. Simply stated, those at risk are men over sixty — and with every decade of advancing age, the risk increases remarkably.

Symptoms of Prostate Cancer

Prostate cancer tends to develop locally for a much longer period of time than does, for example, lung cancer. Because of this, it may cause problems for the patient, or be accessible to diagnosis by physical examination, long before it has spread beyond the prostate gland and is therefore more difficult to treat. A man may notice an increased frequency of urination, an increase in the number of times having to get up at night to urinate, or a certain hesitancy in starting urination. He may sense an urgency to get to the bathroom and then be able to urinate only in small amounts. He will undoubtedly think he has "a prostate problem." Most commonly, in an elderly male with these symptoms, the prostate will have simply enlarged, *unrelated* to cancer. Time is, in this case, certainly on the side of the patient. However, prostate cancers may also cause these symptoms, and the earlier the cancer is diagnosed the greater the chance for cure.

I have a patient, a sturdy man of seventy, who is facing the long arduous prospect of dying from widespread prostate cancer. He had presented himself to a very busy practitioner some two years before he saw me, complaining of "prostate problems." The physician, confronted with hordes of patients in his waiting room and used to similar complaints in elderly men, did not perform a rectal examination, a grave mistake. He gave the patient pills to help him urinate more easily. The patient, because of lack of sophistication and because a rectal examination is a nuisance anyway, accepted this treatment without question.

What might the patient have done at this point instead? He might have said, "I'm worried about prostate cancer."

Or a family member might have accompanied him to his doctor's visit and expressed his or her fears. This kind of advocacy keeps the patient on the team and the doctor on his toes.

Periodically over the ensuing months, he would complain about increasing problems with urination. His medication was increased. Finally, two years later, his family insisted that he get a second opinion. By this time, the cancer was easily felt by the examining rectal finger. Indeed, a layperson could have diagnosed the disease. And, by this time, tests demonstrated that the cancer had spread to the lymph glands in the area and to the man's bones. *The gerbils had already been given run of the palace.* Eradicating them is now almost impossible, but, in the case of prostate cancer, slowing the growth of the cancer cells and providing the patient with a prolonged, useful life, is relatively easy.

Diagnosing prostate cancers is simple. In most cases a rectal examination is all that is required. The palpating finger easily feels the suspicious nodule. If you are an elderly male, and therefore at risk of prostate cancer, and if your physician does not *insist* upon your having an annual rectal examination, *find another physician.*

Treatment of Prostate Cancer

Treatment of prostate cancer in the early stages, before it has spread outside the area of the prostate gland, is highly successful. Both radiation therapy and surgery offer very good chances for cure. It is in your best interests to discuss the options for treatment with your primary physician, a urologist, and an oncologist. Success in treatment of prostate cancer once it has spread beyond the gland will depend upon how aggressive the cancer itself is. Those cancers that are more slowly growing can be checked quite successfully and for long periods of time with hormonal therapy: either through administration of estrogens (female hormones), or by eliminating male hormones through castration. Castration has its psychological problems for the male. But hormonal therapy with estrogens has more significant medical problems associated with it: a higher incidence of blood clots, heart disease, and stroke.

CANCER OF THE UTERUS

Uterine cancer is the last of the common cancers we shall consider. Twenty percent of all cancers afflicting women in America have their origin in the uterus, either in the cervix or in the lining of the uterus, the endometrium. Risk factors for the two cancers of the uterus are different; we shall consider them together.

Risk Factors for Cancer of the Uterus

Cancer of the Cervix:
> Low socioeconomic class
> First intercourse at early age
> Sexual promiscuity
> Large number of pregnancies
> History of estrogen use in mother

Cancer of the Endometrium:
> Obesity
> High blood pressure
> Diabetes
> Use of estrogens

There are important differences about the two cancers arising in the uterus. Cervical cancer most commonly occurs in younger women, whereas cancer of the endometrium occurs more frequently between the ages of fifty and seventy. Cancer of the cervix is neither caused by, nor has any relationship to, the use of oral contraceptives (estrogens). On the contrary, estrogen therapy for relief of menopausal symptoms has a direct relationship to increasing the risk of cancer of the endometrium. Another important difference is in how the diagnosis of each cancer is made. Cervical cancer is almost always without symptoms in its early stages. It is found by routine Pap smear. In contrast, cancer of the endometrium almost always causes vaginal bleeding, *almost always.* In a woman, after menopause, the occurrence of vaginal bleeding should *always* prompt the patient to seek its cause, assuming the worst until proven otherwise. A woman, for example, who has had a normal Pap smear and normal pelvic examination and who develops postmenopausal vaginal bleeding six months later, should immediately go to her doctor to investigate that symptom. A Pap smear will often *not* indicate evidence of *endometrial* cancer even though it is a sensitive test for *cervical* cancer. But selective samplings from within the uterus, called **curettage,** will help in making the diagnosis of endometrial cancer.

Fibroid tumors of the uterus are very common in women after age thirty. These are benign, noncancerous muscle tumors of the uterus and, unless they cause symptoms of pain and/or uncontrolled vaginal bleeding, they can be left alone. Fibroid tumors will *not* develop into cancers.

Screening for Uterine Cancer

What are the best screening maneuvers for early detection of cancers of the uterus? The American Cancer Society recommends Pap smears, pelvic examinations, and rectal examinations at varying frequencies according to age. In our practice, we ask our patients to have *annual* pelvic examinations with rectal examination and with Pap smear. We stress this in our practice because a third malignancy of the female genital system, ovarian cancer, is so rapidly growing and can be found by pelvic examination. It may or may not be cost effective for a woman to have an annual Pap smear and pelvic examination regardless of her age, but it certainly is prudent. I recommend it.

IN SUMMARY: Developments in cancer treatment in the past thirty years have been awesome. The ranges of therapy are many, the options available to the patient complex, and the chances for cure exciting. Proper choice demands proper information. Protect your palace with proper surveillance. Insist upon periodic screening to guard against malignant growth wherever it may occur. Remember:

- That cancers may be curable
- That having a cancer does not mean certain death
- That different cancers behave as differently as the organs from which they arise
- That a thorough periodic physical examination by a physician has great worth and great merit, especially with respect to cancer screening
- That "cost-effective" and tobacco subsidies are a contradiction in terms

A concluding story . . . . A woman went to her doctor and demanded a cancer test. "What kind of cancer test," he inquired? She wanted the kind of cancer test that was talked about on television, the one that checked for cancer of the rectum. "We don't do that here," the doctor said. "Then send me to someone who does it," she answered. "Why do you want it done in the first place," the doctor asked? "Something isn't right," she said. "You're too young for the test, he answered, and besides it's a waste of money."

Because she was stubborn and had a vague sense of disquiet about her palace, she persisted in her search for "the cancer test." Flexible fiberoptic sigmoidoscopy found a polyp in her rectum that had begun to undergo cancerous change. A snip of the polyp and she was cured of her cancer.

May you be as vigilant and as fortunate.

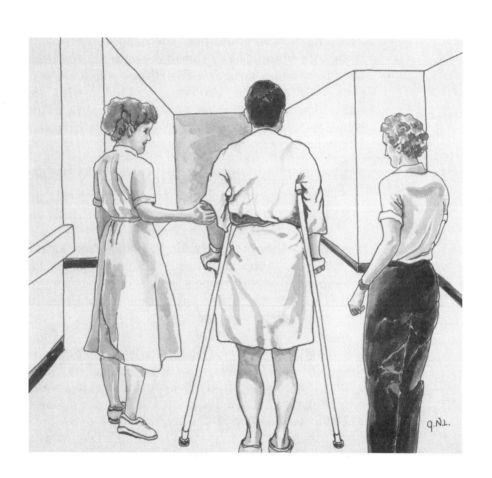

11

Arthritis: Crippled for Life?

*"Some men against rain do carry in their backs
Prognosticating, aching almanacs.
Some by a painful elbow, hip, or knee
Will shrewdly guess what weather's like to be."*

John Taylor
1580-1653

On a makeshift litter, they dragged the old farmer into the emergency room. His wife said that the man, though bedridden for months, shunned doctors and had refused medical attention. He had treated his arthritis with aspirin, worked until he could no more, and then 'took' to bed.

His wrists and knuckles were swollen. His fingers huddled together, drifted to one side, useless. His knees, flexed, swollen, and stiffened, could no longer carry him through his day. He had become a helpless cripple.

We hospitalized the farmer, treated his arthritis with cortisone-like drugs, and summoned the orthopedic surgeons. After several weeks of multiple-drug treatment, reconstructive joint surgery, and intensive physical therapy, he climbed out of bed. Set free from his invalidism, he walked the length of the room and hugged his wife.

Forty years ago, research scientists had searched for just such a patient. Cortisone had recently been synthesized: Clinical investigators were itching to demonstrate its miraculous effect on arthritis with a patient bedridden from rheumatoid arthritis. The researchists gave the cortisone to just such a patient; he too arose from his bed, and the scientists won the Nobel Prize.

CONFUSION OVER ARTHRITIS

But not all arthritis patients experience such disability or such drama. What is arthritis anyway? Is arthritis a *disease* or a *symptom?* Fever is a symptom. Fever may indicate pneumonia, or cancer, or bowel infection, or the flu. No one thinks of fever as a disease, at least not these days. (Three hundred years ago "she died of a fever, did Molly Malone" — but not today, not in our culture, not with our knowledge.)

Nor is a rash a disease. It used to be, in the days when "he had the pox" and physicians didn't know why. But today he can have the pox (a rash) as a *symptom* of syphilis, or chicken pox, or shingles — all three *disease* processes producing as one symptom a rash or "pox."

Joint pain, swelling, and limited motion of joints — these we term arthritis. And arthritis is *also* a symptom of a number of diseases of various causes. The symptom of arthritis indicates the presence of some as yet undefined disease. Because of the various diseases associated with arthritis, great misunderstanding surrounds the painful joint. Since all joint pain does not have the same cause, we need to know which disease is causing the symptom of arthritis before we can treat the disease and predict outcome.

A *second* area of confusion about arthritis: Most kinds of arthritis are diseases of ups and downs, exacerbations and remissions, with pain-free periods occurring unrelated to any form of treatment. It is precisely because of the unpredictable nature of the disease — the long symptom-free periods which may occur, lasting sometimes for months or years — that many *supposed* cures for arthritis are claimed. For example, a patient with arthritis may wear copper bracelets and coincidentally begin a period of remission of the disease, thereby forever convinced that the bracelets control the disease. Moreover, because of these unpredictable ups and downs, standard treatment for arthritis is very difficult to evaluate, requiring continuing study of large numbers of patients with *one* form of arthritis over long periods of time.

A *third* area of confusion: There is great variability in severity of a given form of arthritis among patients suffering from that particular disease. One person with rheumatoid arthritis, for example, may have only stiffness of the fingers and mild swelling of the joints, whereas another patient with the *same* disease will develop severe joint deformity and terrible disability over the same period of time.

One patient I remember, a Mr. F. H., a swashbuckling woodsman, came to my office between shipments of pulp, complaining of painful knuckles. Within three years he was dead. He died of rheumatoid lung disease, one of the uncommon complications of the disease. Another patient, a Mr. T. S., an avid golfer, *with the same disease of rheumatoid arthritis,* has continued to enjoy golf and to live a productive life ten years after the diagnosis of rheumatoid arthritis.

Remember the following points about arthritis:

- Arthritis has many causes, and most forms of arthritis have long, symptom-free periods.
- There is great individual variation in severity of each arthritic disease.
- Most forms of arthritis have no cure.
- There is good, effective therapy for arthritis.

It is no wonder that patients suffering from such a whimsical disease can be so vulnerable to quackery, so prone to frustration. Patients with arthritis are beguiled with a dazzling array of quackery: Charlatans offer magical lotions, bee venoms, manipulative cures, and diet-megavitamin therapy. The money squandered is in the millions, the lives wasted, profound.

RHEUMATOID ARTHRITIS

Rheumatoid arthritis most commonly affects the smaller joints of the body: the hands, the wrists, the feet. Its cause is *unknown*. The disease produces stiffness in the joints, especially after prolonged inactivity, usually in the morning. There is a tenderness of the joints and pain on motion in the involved joints. The tissues and tendons surrounding the affected joints swell. Most commonly, there is simultaneous involvement of the same joint or group of joints on both sides of the body. Most patients with rheumatoid arthritis develop a specific protein in the blood — **rheumatoid factor** — found through blood testing. This rheumatoid factor is not present in normal people nor is it found in the other common forms of arthritis. Later on with rheumatoid arthritis, there may be typical X-ray findings which can aid in the diagnosis. In contrast to most other forms of arthritis, rheumatoid arthritis may have symptoms involving the entire body: so-called constitutional symptoms of fever, fatigue, loss of appetite, and weight loss.

Early in the course of rheumatoid arthritis, the person will have stiffness, joint swelling, and involvement of the small joints in a symmetrical fashion, but no X-ray findings. Usually no rheumatoid factor is found in the blood at this stage. The diagnosis at this point is an educated guess. It is precisely during this uncertain period that many patients may be branded as having rheumatoid arthritis when in fact they do not. It follows therefore that they may believe themselves to be "cured" of a disease they never had — "cured" through the administration of honey and herbs, electromagnetic therapy, or whatever.

A young woman entered our hospital with findings very suggestive of early rheumatoid arthritis. She had acutely painful joints in her hands and fingers with fever, aching in other joints, and a general sense of malaise. We thought at the time that she might have early rheumatoid arthritis, though blood tests for that disease were negative (as they usually are early in the disease process). She embarked on a program of herbs and honey. Her arthritis went away. To this day, she still believes that her health food cured her disease. She may be correct, but we tend to think that she had Lyme arthritis (see below), a self-limited, viral-induced arthritis very similar in its early stages to the early stages of rheumatoid arthritis.

What can the typical patient with rheumatoid arthritis expect? Even though rheumatoid arthritis is thought to be "the crippling kind" of arthritis, in fact only about *ten percent* of patients with the diagnosis become completely incapacitated, and even then only ten to fifteen years after the onset of the disease. *Over fifty percent* of patients with rheumatoid arthritis remain fully employed. *Ten to twenty percent* of patients with rheumatoid arthritis experience an extended period of complete absence of disease symptoms. But patients with the disease who have episodic flare-ups and only partial remissions usually have a gradual progression of deformity and disability. Those few whose disease is unremitting may become completely disabled within a few years of the onset of the disease.

The deformities and the disability are the result of loss of **joint cartilage** — the gristle between the bones —with freezing of the joints, destruction of tendons and ligaments, and subsequent dislocation of joints and deformity. In a few patients with rheumatoid arthritis, the destruction of small arteries can result in skin changes and in organ damage as well.

Although it is difficult to predict the outcome of rheumatoid arthritis, a poor outlook normally results when the patient has one or more of the following:

- Very high amounts of rheumatoid factor in the blood
- Skin changes typical of the disease
- Sustained unremitting disease over a period of a year
- Onset of the disease before age thirty
- Constitutional symptoms, such as fever, fatigue, loss of appetite, weight loss

The natural reactions of a patient with rheumatoid arthritis, with its unpredictable flare-ups and periods of remission, are depression and despair. These patients *do* become desperate, spending over five hundred million dollars per year on arthritis quackery. Because of the nature of the disease, people are vulnerable to "secret formula arthritis cures," "orthomolecular diets," and "miraculous electronic devices." The arthritis victim who has a temporary remission by coincidence at just the moment when he or she is trying some special quackery becomes a believer, or worse, a preaching convert. These patients may even develop the notion that the orthodox medical profession is either ignorant of the disease or deliberately withholding effective therapy for some diabolical purpose or personal gain.

There *is* effective treatment for rheumatoid arthritis, treatment which can alter the course of the disease and diminish the resulting disability. The tragedy is that time and money are wasted on quackery while the joint destruction from the disease continues. A patient with rheumatoid arthritis should view critically anyone who offers special or "secret" formulas, diets, or cures for arthritis. The quack commonly accuses the medical profession of persecuting or misunderstanding the patient and will advertise quick and easy cures. He spurns orthodox medicines as unnecessary poisons to the body. Remember that there are no easy answers for rheumatoid arthritis. *But there are effective therapies.*

Treatment of Rheumatoid Arthritis

Imagine awakening each morning with painful stiffness in every joint. You are all but immobile. Normal household chores seem insurmountable. You have been diagnosed as having early rheumatoid arthritis. You conjure up images of deformities, wheelchairs, and nursing homes. Now imagine that with this disease and these anxieties, your doctor has offered you **aspirin!** With so serious a disease, you think, you certainly need more than aspirin. Any disease is frightening — a disease that persists and is chronic is more so. At this crucial point in the care of an arthritis patient, the well-intentioned but uncommunicative doctor may lose his patient with rheumatoid arthritis to quackery. But the fact is, aspirin *is* effective, inexpensive, available, low in toxicity, and, used correctly, the mainstay of arthritis therapy. It *should* be the first drug prescribed to people with rheumatoid arthritis.

Aspirin Suppresses Inflammation

Many forms of arthritis cause inflammation of joints. The joints swell, as white blood cells attack some as yet unknown agent (as in rheumatoid arthritis), or a known agent (as in gout). In this heat of battle, the white blood cells release toxins of their own. This inflammatory response to the foreign agent, which may be bacteria, viruses, uric acid crystals, or antibodies, injures the body's joint linings and the cartilage and bone as well — the innocent victims of the joint space conflict. Drugs which quiet this inflammation — **anti-inflammatory drugs** — can lessen the damage to these innocent bystanders. Used in proper doses, aspirin is a great anti-inflammatory drug.

Ironically, aspirin's chief shortcoming is its price! People wonder how anything that cheap can be any good. But with large doses of aspirin and high blood levels maintained, aspirin can work wonders in arthritis. People with rheumatoid arthritis need to take eight to twelve tablets of aspirin per day, a dose possibly altered through periodic laboratory determination of aspirin blood levels. With such treatment, joint inflammation usually subsides. Damage to the joints can be spared. The secret of aspirin therapy for rheumatoid arthritis is *to continue treatment even when feeling better.* Inflammation and joint damage are checked only as long as the drug is used. Remember, *there is no cure for rheumatoid arthritis.*

Aspirin Substitutes

Some patients cannot take aspirin. Others tolerate it poorly. Aspirin has its side effects. With high doses, ringing of the ears may occur. This side effect may disappear with a decrease in the dosage. Allergy, heartburn, and stomach ulcers can also be a problem. There are aspirin preparations coated with antacid (Ecotrin and Ascriptin, for example) that may avoid stomach irritation and are just as effective as common aspirin.

Most over-the-counter nonprescription arthritis preparations contain **salicylates,** the active ingredient of aspirin. These proprietary medicines are no more effective than aspirin, but are certainly more costly. (One has to finance the television commercials after all!) Those patients who feel that high cost means better therapy are attracted to these well-packaged items. *They are no better than aspirin.*

For those who simply cannot take aspirin at all, there are *plenty* of substitutes. But a caution about one aspirin substitute: The most commonly used aspirin substitute, acetaminophen (Tylenol, Tempra, Datril) is not anti-inflammatory at all. Acetaminophen will *not* treat arthritis. A whole host of other aspirin substitutes *will* treat arthritis. These drugs, which are of the class called **nonsteroidal anti-inflammatory drugs** and which are listed in Table 11-1, are all similar to aspirin in their anti-inflammatory properties. They are as effective as aspirin. All are far more expensive. Precisely because rheumatoid arthritis is so variable, one indi-

TABLE 11–1 Nonsteroidal Anti-Inflammatory Drugs

Drug	Usual Dosage per day (mg)	Cost of a Month's Treatment
ibuprophen	1800-2400	$13.00
Motrin		25.00
Advil		20.00
Nuprin		19.00
Rufen		16.00
Ibumed		10.00
Ibren		14.00
Ifen		5.00
indomethacin	75-150	12.00
Indocin		40.00
Indameth		14.00
Indocin SR		32.00
fenoprofen	900-2400	28.00
Nalfon		36.00
diclofenac		
Voltaren	100-150	39.00
ketoprophen		
Orudis	150-300	42.00
meclofenamate sodium	600-1600	39.00
Meclomen		50.00
Meclofen		36.00
naproxen		
Naprosyn	500-1000	33.00
naproxen sodium		
Anaprox	500-800	32.00
piroxican		
Feldene	20	47.00
sulindac		
Clinoril	300-400	46.00
tolmetin		
Tolectin	600-1200	32.00

Note: A generic drug is the chemical name of the drug. It is usually cheaper than the trade name for the drug, capitalized in the chart above. A banana is the generic; a Chiquita banana is the trade name.

vidual may respond to one nonsteroidal anti-inflammatory drug and not another. Physician and patient will have to search for the most effective drug in this class.

One nonsteroidal anti-inflammatory drug is not in the list above: phenylbutazone (Butazolidine). This is a potent drug with high toxicity and should no longer be used.

The Patient With Too Many Doctors

Consider a common scenario. A young woman complains to her doctor of pain and swelling of the knuckles. She has generally not been feeling well. She has lost a little weight, has no appetite, sometimes feels feverish, and feels that other joints are stiff and "arthritic." Her physician starts her on high dose aspirin therapy, eight to twelve tablets a day. He measures her aspirin levels in the blood and, on this dosage of aspirin, finds the levels to be within the therapeutic range. Blood testing does not reveal any rheumatoid factor, yet. With the aspirin therapy, her joint inflammation quiets down. Her joints become more mobile, less tender, less painful. She goes back to work and generally feels better.

Now enter the relative, a self-proclaimed expert on arthritis! This relative, as the scenario commonly goes, has heard of a "new" drug for arthritis, usually one of the newer nonsteroidal anti-inflammatory drugs. "Your physician is mistreating you, giving you *just* aspirin," so the relative advises. "You should be on this new drug." The relative mentions Feldene, Motrin, or one of the other drugs on the list above. The patient begins to question her doctor's judgment. Why wasn't this new drug started? Why am I being given *common* aspirin? Does my doctor know what he's doing? And so the patient begins the search for an "arthritis specialist." What has happened? The young patient with rheumatoid arthritis may well find a very capable, knowledgable **rheumatologist** (arthritis specialist), but because of mistrust, will needlessly have discarded her primary doctor.

Gold Therapy for Rheumatoid Arthritis

Chemical compounds containing gold are anti-inflammatory. They are often very effective in treating rheumatoid arthritis. If aspirin and nonsteroidal anti-inflammatory drugs fail to provide remission of disease, gold compounds are often tried. In many cases, such gold compounds can lead to long-term remission of disease. These gold-containing chemicals may be given either by injection or by mouth. Injection with gold compounds for rheumatoid arthritis is inconvenient, expensive, but nevertheless *usually preferred*. Injection in the doctor's office affords the patient better surveillance for drug toxicity. The injections are given weekly at first, for the first ten to twelve weeks of therapy, and then are given monthly for an indefinite period. The response to gold injections is slow, with the benefit occurring over months, and certainly not overnight. Frequent blood and urine testing is *absolutely mandatory* for the rheumatoid patient getting gold therapy. If not recognized early, the side effects from gold can be fatal. It is because of the need to test for side effects that I demand that my patients with rheumatoid arthritis who receive gold therapy get it by injection in the office, where I can check them for possible toxicity.

The pill form of gold therapy is just as effective, but one runs the danger of a patient who takes the bit in his mouth: He takes the pill, avoids the doctor and puts himself at risk. Testing for drug side effects doesn't get done.

Despite the expense and the inconvenience, gold therapy is a very effective form of therapy for rheumatoid arthritis — seventy percent of rheumatoid patients respond favorably to it.

Other Therapies for Rheumatoid Disease

Plaquenil and *penicillamine* are two very potent drugs used to treat rheumatoid arthritis. Their side effects can be serious; these drugs should never be used in a cavalier manner. *Cortisone* preparations (prednisone, dexamethasone, Decadron, Deltasone, and others) suppress inflammation quite dramatically and relieve the suffering of rheumatoid arthritis in a miraculous way. For arthritis sufferers and especially for those with rheumatoid arthritis, cortisone preparations are true miracle drugs if properly used. The temptation is to use the drug too often and in great quantities. This is a siren's song. *Unrestrained treatment with cortisone-type drugs can be worse than the disease itself.* Cortisone weakens resistance to infection, causes thinning of the tissues and easy bruising, fat deposits, severe mental reactions, high blood sugars and diabetes, high blood pressure, and marked thinning of the bone. Cortisone may cause cataracts, muscle weakness, high cholesterol, and in some cases even bone destruction. Used judiciously and under the supervision of a physician, cortisone can be a God-send. Used indiscriminately, it can be a disaster.

The Beekeeper

I have an elderly patient with arthritis who keeps bees. He likes to "get stung at least once a day." He has learned over the years that, for some reason unknown to him, the transient discomfort of a bee sting is markedly outweighed by the relief it affords him from his arthritis. What happens to him on a daily basis is that the bee sting excites a complex hormonal reaction in his body, which in turn causes an increase in cortisone production by his body. And this increase in cortisone production relieves his arthritis!

Treating arthritis is tricky business. The cookbook, computerized approach seldom works. Usually combinations of drugs are necessary, together with physical therapy, exercises, rest, reconstructive surgery, and, most of all, emotional support. There is no cure for rheumatoid arthritis, but the physician who cares and who knows what he is doing can help immensely. He need *not* be an arthritis specialist. He had better not be a quack. When you find a physician you trust to treat your arthritis, stay with him or her. Don't shop around. And certainly, avoid needless expense, patent medicines, quacks, and gimmickery.

OSTEO-ARTHRITIS

Osteoarthritis, or degenerative joint disease, is the arthritis of advancing age. All of us develop this kind of arthritis if we live long enough. It is the most common form of arthritis. Thirty-seven percent of *all* adults and ninety-seven percent of those over the age of sixty have this form of arthritis. Osteoarthritis is the result of simple wear and tear on the joints. Therefore, the joints most commonly used, those physically burdened in life, will be most commonly affected.

The hips, knees, spine, and outermost joints of the fingers suffer frequent wear and tear and so are prone to osteoarthritis, whereas osteoarthritis tends to spare the wrists, elbows, shoulders, ankles, and the bases of the fingers. (This is distinct from rheumatoid arthritis which commonly affects these joints. See Figure 11-1A.)

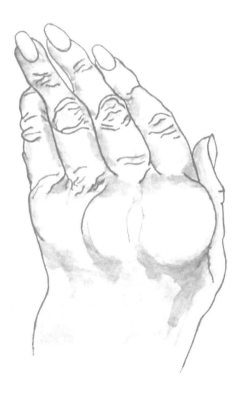

FIGURE 11–1A   An Example of Rheumatoid Arthritis of the Hands

Osteoarthritis differs from rheumatoid arthritis in another way as well. There is *seldom* swelling, redness, or increased heat — the inflammation we have talked about — in the joint affected with osteoarthritis, and there are *never* the constitutional symptoms one finds in rheumatoid disease — symptoms of weight loss, fatigue, or involvement of internal organs.

Continued use of a joint eventually wears away the gristle of the joint-space, called the cartilage tissue and *synovium*. The joint loses its elastic cushion and its lubrication. The cartilage frays. Bone begins to grate upon bone. The result is pain. If the process becomes severe, the joint becomes distorted and markedly restricted in motion. This constitutes the disease osteoarthritis. It is a degeneration of joints, hence called **degenerative joint disease.** One sign of the disease is the bony enlargement at the ends of the fingers, as seen in the hands in Figure 11-1B. Some people are more prone to this joint wear and tear than others and may develop osteoarthritis as early as age forty. The disease also seems to be more common in women than in men. Trauma to a particular joint may hasten the development of osteoarthritis in that joint.

Physical therapy and exercise can help tremendously in preventing immobility of joints and in preserving function when joints are affected by osteoarthritis. Treating obesity is critical in the treatment of osteoarthritis — losing weight lessens the burden on weightbearing joints. Aspirin and the nonsteroidal anti-inflammatory drugs already discussed can be very effective for pain relief.

Surgery for Osteoarthritis

Joint reconstruction, especially replacement of the arthritic hips and knees, is a common procedure today. Candidates for this surgery are generally patients over sixty who have good circulation in the extremities, are not terribly obese and, because hip reconstruction is especially stressful, are generally healthy otherwise. When is reconstructive surgery for hip and knee arthritis indicated? Your physician should consider recom-

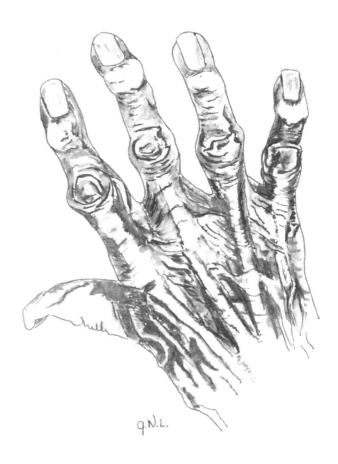

FIGURE 11–1B   An Example of Osteoarthritis of the Hand

mending such surgery to you if you experience any of the following:

- You have pain in the affected joint at night.
- You cannot continue with your job.
- Medicines do not alleviate the pain.
- You cannot enjoy your day.
- You have difficulty with climbing stairs.
- You have difficulty getting into a car.
- You cannot drive.

- You cannot tie your shoes or clip your toenails (because of hip disease).
- You can no longer make love (because of painful hip disease).

GOUT

Gout is an arthritis caused by chemical imbalance. The chemical, uric acid, is a waste product normally found in the blood. In patients with gout, because of an inability to excrete the uric acid or because of an over-production of it, the concentration of uric acid rises above normal. The excess uric acid crystals settle out in the tissues, joints, and sometimes even in the kidneys, much as does excess salt in brine. The crystals in the joint space incite an attack by white blood cells. As with rheumatoid arthritis, inflammation in the joint begins. Arthritis is the result. Occasionally the crystals deposit in the kidneys, damaging those organs and leading to kidney stones.

Consider this classical description of gout by a seventeenth century physician suffering from one of his own gout attacks:

> *The victim goes to bed and sleeps in good health. About two o'clock in the morning he is awakened by severe pain in the great toe (more rarely in the heel, ankle, or instep). The pain is like that of a dislocation, and yet the parts feel as if cold water were poured over them. Then follow chills and shivers and a little fever. The pain, which was at first moderate, becomes more intense. With its intensity, the chills and shivers increase. Now it is a violent stretching and tearing of the ligaments — now it is a gnawing pain, and now a pressure and tightening. So exquisite and lively, meanwhile, is the feeling of the part affected, that it cannot bear the weight of the bedclothes nor the jar of a person walking in the room. The night is passed in torture,*

sleeplessness, turning of the part affected and perpetual changing of posture.

Myths About Gout

There are many misconceptions about gout. A high uric acid level does not necessarily indicate gout. Twice as many people have abnormally high levels of uric acid in the blood as ever develop gout. Nor does a sore toe together with the finding of a high blood test for uric acid *necessarily* mean one has gout. Diagnosing gout is more complicated than drawing a blood test. Needling the joint to withdraw the crystals, collecting the urine for uric acid, and sometimes X-raying the joint are often required for diagnosis. Still, many patients suffering from *osteoarthritis* are mistakenly labeled as having *gout* because of a single blood test. Since treatment of gout is different from that for osteoarthritis, distinguishing between the two forms of arthritis is crucial.

A second misconception about gout concerns diet. Although diet control can be important in the treatment of the disease, a single dietary indiscretion will not cause a gout attack. Fasting, in fact, is more likely to do so. There is also the notion, equally false, that wealthy people with splendid diets are the only people who get gout. Membership in the middle class, with its less spectacular dietary fare, does not protect you against gout.

Treatment of Gout

Gout cannot be cured, but the drugs available today to control the disease do it so well that kidney damage is avoided and acute arthritis rarely if ever occurs. Remember, gout medicine must be taken for life. Too often patients take the medicines for a few months and then, believing themselves cured, stop the drugs . *Colchicine* and *indomethacin* both treat an acute gout attack very effectively. With these drugs, a gout attack can usually be checked within twenty-four hours. Allopurinol (Zyloprim) and probenecid (Benemid) lower the blood levels of uric acid and will prevent future attacks. They can prevent kidney damage as well. Allopurinol and probenecid are of no use in the acute attack of gout, nor are they of any use in other forms of arthritis. Curiously, *aspirin* can make gout worse. Aspirin prevents the body's elimination of uric acid and can increase the blood levels of uric acid in the gouty patient. Knowing which form of arthritis one has is extremely important!

A Backwoods Entrepreneur

In their childhood years, my sons grew by one shoe size about every three weeks. I learned of an inexpensive place to buy shoes. A man of the woods, I discovered, regularly drove a truck to Boston, purchased huge lots of shoes wholesale and trucked them back to the woods. There, he sold them from the shacks and mobile homes he had placed among the pine. Low overhead was the idea. One day, after a lot of back and forth dirt-road-driving, I found his place. His wife was bustling about waiting on customers while the entrepreneur himself sat among the boxes, immobile and in obvious pain. He had, he said, excruciating pain in a big toe and in his right elbow. This seemed to come and go, haunting him over the years. He figured it was 'arthritis.' I asked to see the elbow. It was flaming red and swollen. He held it out to me gingerly as if begging me not to touch it, not wanting me to inflict pain. I quickly looked at the cartilage of his ears and found what I had suspected might be there: deposits of uric acid crystals in small lumps under the skin, called **tophi.** The man had **tophaceous gout,** a disease miserably incurable in Henry VIII's time, but eminently treatable today. I drove back to town and got him some samples of indomethacin. In twenty-four hours he was asymptomatic. Several days later, still on the indomethacin, he began taking allopurinol as well. He has continued his medication to this day. His tophi have disappeared and his gout attacks have never returned. *And I have never wanted for shoes since.*

POLYMYALGIA RHEUMATICA

Polymyalgia rheumatica, a sort of "rheumatism," is not really an arthritis, but certainly deserves mention here.

Not an uncommon disease, it is found almost exclusively in elderly patients. *It is often under-diagnosed.* This disease affects chiefly the muscles of the shoulders and hips, producing a morning stiffness, pain on motion, lethargy, and some weight loss. The patient, typically elderly, often volunteers a complaint of soreness in the shoulders, hips, or low back. He or she complains of "trouble getting around." The physician may or may not find some muscle tenderness, but finds no evidence of arthritis per se. This is a disease of *muscles* rather than *joints*. What is so potentially devastating about this disease is this: In as many as forty percent of patients with this muscle disorder, the arteries supplying the retinas can become inflamed. Sudden blindness can result. Pain, headache, and tenderness in the temples can also signal the presence of polymyalgia rheumatica. A simple blood test, the sedimentation rate, cinches the diagnosis. The disease responds dramatically to low doses of cortisone-like drugs. Blindness can always be prevented by early treatment.

A Baffling Case

An elderly woman was referred to a psychiatrist. Her family had noted some changes in her behavior: She acted vague, her memory frequently failed her, and sometimes she did not quite make sense. The psychiatrist could not make a definite diagnosis beyond labeling her as "possibly early dementia." She began to complain of pain in her jaw when eating. It pained her a great deal, she complained, even to comb her hair. She had a continual headache in her temples. Her physician-daughter took a careful history. Yes, the elderly lady admitted, she had rheumatism as well. Her shoulders ached continually, as did her hips and thighs. She was stiff in the morning, had no energy, and had lost some weight.

Her daughter obtained a sedimentation rate. It was markedly elevated. A biopsy of the artery near her temple demonstrated inflammation in that artery, the "temporal arteritis" so often associated with polymyalgia rheumatica, and so often leading to sudden blindness. *The woman was started on low doses of cortisone and was dramatically cured.*

LESS COMMON FORMS OF ARTHRITIS

Ankylosing spondylitis is an uncommon disease. It is an arthritis of the spine, with other joints of the body occasionally becoming inflamed as well. It is usually not as crippling as rheumatoid arthritis, tends to run in families, and affects primarily young males. It is so common in people with certain types of tissue protein, called HLA B-27, that a test for this protein in a patient with back pain virtually makes the diagnosis. Treatment is primarily symptomatic: physical therapy, weight control, and anti-inflammatory drugs.

Systemic lupus erythematosus usually strikes young women. The arthritis in lupus is very similar to that of rheumatoid arthritis. Fever, rash, and kidney problems are more frequent in lupus, however, than in rheumatoid arthritis. Many cases of lupus are mild and can be treated with brief courses of cortisone-like drugs and anti-inflammatory agents. But the disease is chronic and can be potentially life-threatening. It can be difficult to treat, and requires an internist or rheumatologist well versed in its treatment for supervision of care.

Likewise, **scleroderma** is uncommon and as difficult to treat. Scleroderma produces a rheumatoid-like arthritis as well as hardening of the skin, various organ abnormalities and, commonly, whitening of the fingers upon exposure to cold. *A caution!* Many people may have whitening of the digits upon cold exposure — so-called **Raynaud's phenomenon** — without ever having scleroderma. As with lupus, many cases of scleroderma are mild in form, but the disease can be as devastating.

Infectious arthritis is common. The joint space becomes infected with bacteria. Swelling, tenderness, pain, and limitation of motion, *usually in one joint only,* are the result. The bacteria gain access to the joint through contiguous trauma or a break in the skin, or sometimes through a blood-borne infection, most notably with gonorrhea. To diagnose infectious arthritis properly, the joint should be aspirated. With local anesthesia, a needle is placed in the joint space and the joint fluid withdrawn and examined for presence of infection and inflammation. Joint infection is curable if it is recognized promptly and not confused with other forms of joint inflammation.

LYME ARTHRITIS

One form of infectious arthritis deserves emphasis these days. Lyme disease is now the most common insect-borne illness occurring in the United States. Its original focus in Lyme, Connecticut, is expanding rapidly. The bacterium, a spirochete, is transmitted to the human host through the bite of the northern deer tick. Typically, in the affected individual the bite produces an intense rash at the site of the tick bite. Following this, there may be a more generalized rash. The arthritis of Lyme disease most commonly affects the large joints, the knees in particular, with joint inflammation: swelling, redness, pain, and increased heat. In addition, the patient with Lyme disease may suffer from headache, stiff neck, fatigue — all of the signs suggestive of a meningitis. Heart problems and liver problems can also occur.

Wherever deer are abundant in New England, Lyme disease is endemic. In addition to the deer population, the spirochete causing Lyme disease infects the mouse population as well. The deer tick, feeding on the mice and deer, in turn becomes infected with the Lyme disease spirochete. Domestic pets — dogs and cats —then carry the deer ticks inside to the potential human hosts.

A simple blood test can diagnose the disease. Early antibiotic therapy is curative. If the diagnosis is missed, a chronic arthritis can result, as can the other organ damage mentioned above.

If you live in the Northeast, and if you develop a localized red rash, *especially* on the extremity, and especially if associated with a tick bite, think of Lyme disease and see your physician immediately. This kind of arthritis is curable.

A Brief Quiz   A sailor from Newport, Rhode Island, seeks medical
attention for a painful arthritis of his big toe. He gives a
history. He has a girl in every port. He does a lot of
jumping and banging around on the ship. He has spent
some time walking in the woods in Rhode Island when
he is on shore leave. His father and grandfather had
gout. He *could* have

> Lyme disease
> Gout
> Osteoarthritis from trauma
> Infectious arthritis from gonorrhea
> All of the above
> (Answer below)

SUMMARY

- Remember that arthritis is a *symptom* of disease
  and not a disease itself.
- Diagnosing the various types of arthritis can be
  very difficult indeed. A painful toe may indicate
  gout, infection from gonorrhea, osteoarthritis, rheumatoid arthritis, or Lyme disease. You cannot be
  expected to make a distinction among these various
  diseases, but you should be aware of the many
  diseases which must be considered.
- Medicines can be dramatically effective in arthritis
  but must not be used in shotgun fashion without a
  diagnosis. There is no *one* medicine to treat all
  forms of arthritis.
- Remember that aspirin can help rheumatoid arthritis but can aggravate gout.
- Be aware of the possible dangers of drug therapy,
  that is, of the toxicity of drugs. In some cases the
  side effects from drugs can be worse than the
  disease itself.
- Remember that most forms of arthritis are chronic
  and do not have a cure, although effective therapy
  is available.
- Remember that obesity aggravates the burden of
  diseased weightbearing joints in all forms of

arthritis, and that extreme obesity can itself cause osteoarthritis of the weightbearing joints.

- An informed patient helps his or her physician by providing accurate information, *a good history,* to assist the physician in making a diagnosis. But, as is in the case of our sailor above, *all of the diagnoses listed are possible,* and it remains for the astute clinician to do proper testing to arrive at a proper diagnosis.
- An informed patient can better assess his or her medical care by judging how the doctor listens and what the doctor considers when confronting a case of arthritis.
- As with any disease, the informed patient with arthritis becomes an aware patient, better able to participate in his or her own medical care.

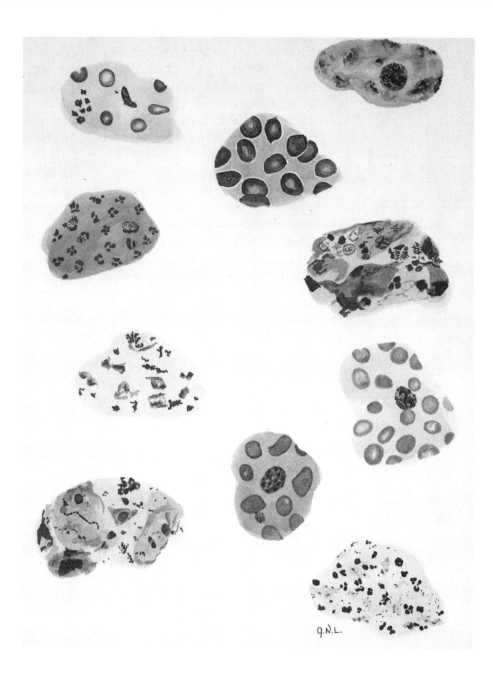

12

Common Infections

"What timid man does not avoid contact with the sick, fearing lest he contract a disease so near?"

Ovid (43 B.C. - 17 A.D.)

THE NATURE OF INFECTION

To understand infectious diseases, we should return to the palace metaphor of Chapter Ten. The palace is a metaphor for the human body. For purposes of our discussion, the most vital contents of the palace are its family, its pets, and its palace guards. The plant life within the palace is expendable. (This is true also with bacteria — plant life — within the human body.)

In our cancer metaphor some of the *animal* tissue (the gerbils) reproduced uncontrollably and threatened the very life of the palace. With infectious diseases, the palace is threatened by unchecked growth of *plants* rather than animals. If there is no effort to contain the plants, they may choke the palace's kitchen or ventilation system. By interfering with the function of such vital parts of the palace, they may bring about the destruction of the entire palace itself. Extending the metaphor to the human body, recall that bacteria are plants and that certain bacteria, pneumococci, may infect the body's ventilation system (the lungs), causing pneumonia. Untreated, this pneumonia, a plant-like infection of the lungs, can result eventually in killing the body.

Remember also that successful treatment depends upon essential differences between the normal inhabitants of the palace and its unwanted invaders. The greater the differences between palace resident and unwanted guest, the more simple and less toxic the treatment. But the more similar the invading guest is to the palace residents — the more the unwanted guest "looks" like the inhabitants of the palace — the more difficult it becomes to treat an invasion, whether it is infection or cancer. It is very important to keep this in mind: Namely, *that treatment depends upon essential differences between host (yourself) and invader (infection)*. If you remember this one point, you can, with the material in this chapter, begin to understand why antibiotics cannot solve every problem of infectious disease, why treatment of the common cold must rely upon the body's own defenses (given our present state of knowledge), and why medical science has thus far found it impossible to treat or prevent infection with the AIDS virus.

The Shotgun and the Laser

In the United States, most common infections are caused by plant-like organisms. Worldwide, it is a different story. Two billion people, for example, are infected with two species of parasitic worms. Six hundred million people are infected by malaria, caused by a microscopic animal-parasite. But for our discussion here, we shall limit our analysis to infections caused by plant life: *viruses* and *bacteria*. And though there are other, esoteric methods of fighting infection, we will examine here the two most common defenses, reliance upon the body's own defense mechanisms and the use of antibiotics. A comparison of the two approaches to infection — **host defenses** versus **antibiotics** — is analogous to comparing a finely focused laser to the spray of buckshot from a shotgun. Antibiotics are like the shotgun, often killing the intended invader, but usually also killing harmless bacteria, innocent bystanders, as well. In contrast, host defenses — the body's infection-fighting white blood cells along with its own antibody system — can be likened to a finely tuned laser. The host defenses are finely focused and accurately attack the infecting agent in question without killing any innocent bystanders. If you can understand the use of antibiotics and its shortcomings, and if you can grasp the concept of the body's own immune system — its white blood cells and antibodies — and its chief threat, AIDS infection, you will then have a good working knowledge of infectious disease in general.

ANTIBIOTICS- A PANACEA?

No prescription drug is more often misused than the antibiotic. There is more confusion surrounding the proper use of antibiotics than there is in any other area of medicine. Patients, when deprived of antibiotics they think necessary, sometimes feel that a physician deliberately withholds from them an available cure.

This attitude is understandable. Only forty or fifty years ago in the pre-antibiotic era, life expectancy was much shorter than it is now, largely because of infectious disease. Young people routinely died of pneumonias. Venereal diseases resulted in sterility, insanity, and sometimes even a slow, agonizing death. Children with simple ear infections died of complicating meningitis. Mankind was literally plagued with bacterial infections.

Then, with one of the greatest discoveries in history, a simple mold was found to produce a substance poisonous to other plants (bacteria). This miraculous substance, penicillin, was isolated and, together with sulfonamides, ushered in the antibiotic era.

These two drugs, penicillin and sulfa, gave every appearance of cure-alls. They controlled and cured many of the previously lethal bacterial infections plaguing us. In the early days of the antibiotic era, penicillin and sulfa were used for virtually every disease, infectious or not, in an attempt to achieve cure.

Over the past forty years, our experience with antibiotics has taught us a great deal about infectious disease:

- We have found other antibiotics far more effective than penicillin and sulfonamides to treat certain infections.
- We have seen bacteria develop resistance to antibiotics to which they were formerly sensitive.
- We have found antibiotics powerless against the whole host of infectious diseases caused by viruses.
- We have learned that certain bacteria residing within us are beneficial and that killing them off with antibiotics can in fact cause problems.
- We are now plagued with a distressingly large list of diseases actually *caused* by antibiotic use.
- Finally, we have learned that no disease can be cured by the use of antibiotics alone.

Almost all infections in our area of the world are caused by bacteria or by viruses. With some minor exceptions, the microscopic plants called bacteria are either killed or controlled by administration of antibiotics. Species of bacteria cause impetigo (an infectious rash common in children), some pneumonias, gonorrhea, bladder infections, some cases of diarrhea, and certain kinds of spinal meningitis, as well as a large list of other infectious diseases. **Viruses** are small bits of chromosome material encased by a protein envelope. Whereas bacteria can be seen with a microscope, viruses are too small to be seen with a common light microscope. (The electron microscope can visualize virus particles). *Viruses are unaffected by antibiotics.* Viruses cause a whole host of infections, some of which include shingles, chicken pox, poliomyelitis, some pneumonias, some venereal infections, many kinds of diarrhea, certain forms of meningitis, and AIDS.

Just as viruses are unaffected by treatment with antibiotics, so certain bacteria may be unaffected by one particular antibiotic. For example, certain kinds of pneumonias and meningitis caused by bacteria will not be treated by penicillin.

Certain principles follow from this information:

- Viral infections are not always easily distinguished from bacterial infections (a pneumonia may be due to either type of infection, virus or bacteria).
- Viruses are unaffected by antibiotics.
- When treating bacterial infections, there is a right drug for each bug.
- It is important, therefore, to distinguish bacterial from viral infections and as important to identify which bacterium is causing the infection, if in fact the infection is bacterial.

Problems with Antibiotic Use

Too often, these principles of infectious disease are forgotten in favor of a shotgun approach to infection. Broad spectrum antibiotics, capable of killing a wide variety of species of bacteria, are somtimes used in huge doses to treat a presumed bacterial infection as yet undefined. The idea is that "if it's bacterial, I'll be able to kill it with this big, powerful, expensive antibiotic in huge doses, and if it's viral, well it doesn't matter anyway."

Such an approach has many potential dangers. *First,* the infection may not be treated at all, but the patient, gaining a false sense of security from the use of the antibiotics, feels that some good is being done. A case report:

Stephanie, age 2, enters an emergency room in near coma. Five days earlier, her doctor began treating her ear infection with penicillin (a wrong choice of drug in this case). Her fever continued. She became more drowsy and, with extension of the infection from the ear to the coverings of the brain, developed meningitis. Her parents delayed further medical attention despite her worsening condition because of their assumption that penicillin, a presumed panacea, would eventually take care of the problem. The child's treatment was delayed and she nearly died because of it.

Second, the administration of antibiotics always raises the possibility of bacterial superinfection. Simply stated, a superinfection is a new, superimposed bacterial infection which can result from antibiotic use. Just as nature abhors a vacuum, she also rushes in to repopulate a sterile environment. Hence, a woman may take ampicillin for a bladder infection. The ampicillin treats the offending infection but also kills off the bacteria normally populating her vagina, which then becomes repopulated with yeast organisms. A vaginal yeast infection results: a superimposed complicating infection.

Third, the use of antibiotics may promote the development of resistance of bacteria to those antibiotics. For example, over the years, with repeated use of penicillin to treat gonorrhea, gonorrhea bacteria have become far less sensitive to penicillin.

A *fourth problem* with antibiotic use is the potential for toxicity. Patients routinely get diarrhea from antibiotic use — a mild side effect. On the other hand, permanent staining of teeth in children inappropriately treated with tetracyclines can result — a much more serious side effect. And, side effects can be lethal: chloramphenicol (Chloromycetin) is an antibiotic which can destroy the bone marrow.

Nor should we neglect the expense involved in antibiotic use. Some of the newer antibiotics cost over a dollar a pill and a seven to ten day course of medication might cost thirty to fifty dollars when in fact a far less expensive antibiotic would treat the infection as well.

An example will illustrate this as well as a few other points:

A physician calls the infectious disease consultant. "I would like you to see a patient of mine. I've just admitted her. She had a cough a couple of weeks ago and I put her on Vibramycin. Now, that pill is over a dollar a dose and I figured it would take care of her cough. She's gotten worse and needs oxygen. Her chest X-ray shows bilateral pneumonias. I need your help."

The infectious disease consultant finds a very sick young woman, whose lungs are infected by a common bacterium resistant to the antibiotic Vibramycin. The patient is coughing up large amounts of infected phlegm. The phlegm is prepared for the microscope as well as being cultured on appropriate nutrient media which encourage the bacteria to grow. Chemical staining of the phlegm gives the infectious disease consultant an idea of the type of infection causing the pneumonia. From this quick test, the consultant can choose an appropriate antibiotic to treat the patient while awaiting specific identification and sensitivities from the cultures.

In retrospect, what should the strategy have been? What should you be aware of as accepted standard procedure? Before treating any bacterial infection with antibiotics, cultures should usually be taken. This means that when there is a bacterial infection, samples of the infected material, whether obtained from a throat swab because of a throat infection, sputum collection because of presumed pneumonia, or urine collection because of a bladder infection — such samples are used to inoculate nutrient media so that the offending bacteria will grow and can be identified. This is the way your physician learns which antibiotics to use in treating a bacterial infection. A patient suffering from infection therefore *should be aware that the taking of cultures is usually a most important first maneuver.* There are, of course, exceptions. In a first time bladder infection, for example, it may not always be necessary to insist that a woman get a urine culture before taking antibiotics. Almost certainly, such an infection will be sensitive to one of the penicillins or sulfonamides and can be treated successfully.

Treating Untreatable Infections

Too frequently, antibiotics are misused in treating infections, especially when being administered for viral infections which, as we know, do *not* respond to antibiotics. When efforts are not made to distinguish a viral infection from a bacterial infection or when it is assumed that a viral illness is caused by a bacterium when it is not, antibiotics may be misused. Often this type of antibiotic misuse occurs when a physician acquiesces to patients' demands. As is true with politics and television, in medicine patients are sometimes given what they want rather than what they need. Quite commonly, a patient will even shop around to find a doctor who will prescribe antibiotics when they are requested and who will prescribe them over the phone for any presumed infection. The patient then assumes that he or she has found a "good" doctor. But this misuse of antibiotics only exposes the patient to any of the possible consequences listed above. And, as you should now know, *the length of a viral illness will not be altered one bit by the use of antibiotics.*

Antibiotics are often used to treat a fever under the mistaken assumption that fever necessarily means infection. As we know from the arthritis chapter, fever may be a manifestation of arthritis, bowel inflammation, some cancers, or a whole host of other non-infectious diseases. And even when fever is due to infection, most often that infection will be viral anyway and therefore untreatable with antibiotics. *Fever should never be treated with antibiotics until it has been proven that a bacterial infection is the cause of the fever.*

Improper Dosage of Antibiotics

People often stop taking antibiotics when they begin to feel better, mistakenly assuming they are "cured." Taking antibiotics for too short a period may, instead of curing the person of infection, encourage the emergence of resistent organisms which will prove only more difficult to treat. In the case of certain streptococcal infections, for example in strep throat, ten full days of the appropriate antibiotic are necessary to prevent the complications of rheumatic fever and nephritis. Remember this: *Symptoms* of infection are caused when a very large number of bacteria has invaded the host. An inappropriately short course of antibiotics in inappropriately low doses may kill some or even most of the organisms but leave behind enough bacteria to reinitiate the infectious illness once the antibiotic is stopped.

Returning to our palace metaphor, let's say it another way: The palace's ventilation system might become threatened by exuberant growth of plants therein. Using an herbicide to kill most, but not all, of the plants will result only in temporary relief of the threat. If some plants are allowed to remain, those plants will reproduce and multiply, eventually threatening the ventilation system again, and quite possibly this time the plants will be resistant to the herbicide previously used.

Failure to Discontinue Antibiotics After Side Effects Occur

Not uncommonly, antibiotics can precipitate an allergic reaction. Patients have a common misconception about this point. Since they have never reacted to a given antibiotic, they assume that they cannot be allergic to that antibiotic, *ever*. Remember: It takes *experience* by the body's immune system to render a person allergic to a given drug. That is the whole basis for the immunizations we will discuss below. That is the basis for allergy as well. Such allergic reactions can run the whole gamut from simple rash to death from shock.

Antibiotics can cause fever as well. If this is not recognized, the antibiotic might be continued under the mistaken assumption that the fever is due to infection rather than to medication. There are other side effects from antibiotics as well, including seizure, sore throat, and massive bleeding problems. Anytime a new complaint, problem, or illness arises *after* taking a drug, antibiotic or otherwise, you should always assume that the new problem is a side effect of the drug. Otherwise, in some instances, failure to stop a drug when side effects occur can be lethal.

Self-Treatment with Leftovers

Just as patients often discontinue antibiotics as soon as they begin to feel better, "thrifty" patients will also save the remainder of the antibiotic pills for the next infection. At the first sign of a cough or scratchy sore throat, the leftover antibiotic is used. The mistake is compounded; not only was the first infection improperly treated, so also is the second infection, both by inappropriate use of antibiotics in inappropriate doses and because antibiotic use *before* cultures are taken will render subsequent cultures useless.

Avoiding Needless Expense

As mentioned above, antibiotics can be expensive; the most expensive antibiotic is not always the most appropriate. Let's look at a simple example. A woman presents with a simple bladder infection. It is a first-time infection. Her physician cultures her urine appropriately and then might prescribe any one of five or six common antibiotics, all *equally* effective in treating her bladder infection. As shown in the table below, the cost of appropriate therapy varies greatly.

If he prescribes:	*The cost will be:*
Gantrisin	$5.99
ampicillin	5.69
Septra or Bactrim	9.69
Keflex (brand)	26.69
Keflex (generic)	16.99
Vibramycin (brand)	43.99
Vibramycin (generic)	9.99

These are approximate retail costs for one week of appropriate therapy. Avoid needless expense.

COMMON BACTERIAL INFECTIONS

Urinary Tract Infections

Bacterial infections of the bladder and kidneys are much more common in women than in men. This is because the female urethra is much shorter than the male urethra and thus allows easier passage of bacteria into the bladder. Also, the female urethra is anatomically close to the vagina, which can in turn harbor organisms potentially infective to the urinary tract.

A woman with an uncomplicated bacterial infection of the bladder will complain of symptoms of bladder irritation. She will have pain on urination, will have to urinate more frequently, and, commonly, such urination will be in small amounts. There will be an urgency to urinate. Occasionally there may be some blood in the urine, but chills and fever most often will be absent. Because these symptoms can also be the result of a vaginal infection, an inspection of the urine, called a **urinalysis,** is often done with such symptoms.

If the urinalysis shows that the urine is not infected, there cannot be a bladder infection.

Vaginal infection should be suspected instead.

If the urinalysis indicates a urinary tract infection, some of the urine is sent to the bacteriology laboratory for cultures. A short course of antibiotics is begun while awaiting cultures.

Should the cultures show the organism responsible for the infection is resistant to the chosen antibiotic, treatment will then be changed. If treatment is already appropriate, it is extended. For a simple, first-infection type of bladder infection, it is entirely appropriate for it to be treated with a single, large dose of antibiotic instead of the well-proven traditional seven- to ten-day course more commonly used.

Occasionally, women will have repeated bladder infections. The following reasons could be the cause:

- An inclination toward a full bladder
- Wiping back to front after a bowel movement, which can colonize the vagina with potentially infective organisms, which in turn gain access to the urethra
- Irritation to the urethra and bladder during sexual intercourse (urinating after intercourse will avoid this cause of recurrent infection)
- Some structural abnormality of the bladder or kidneys (improper emptying of the bladder or retention of some urine will predispose to infection)
- Diabetes mellitus

A good rule to follow is this:

Any woman who has more than two bladder infections in one year should have a more complete investigation for possible secondary cause.

Excluding the existence of diabetes mellitus or a practice of sexual intercourse with a full bladder, such a woman should see a urologist to look for structural problems that may be causing the repeated infections.

Women with recurrent urinary tract infections should be treated with a traditional seven- to ten-day course of antibiotics. If, after investigation, no apparent cause can be found for recurrent urinary tract infections, it may be well-advised for a woman to take a *small* preventative dose of antibiotic every day, indefinitely.

Occasionally, a kidney may become infected when the bladder infection ascends through the drainage system from the bladder to the kidney or when the infection becomes blood-borne. Almost always, a patient with a kidney infection will have chills and fever together with pain in the flank. This is *always* a serious infection and usually requires hospitalization and administration of intravenous antibiotics.

Strep Throat

Sore throat is a very common complaint and it is most often caused by infection. Although most throat infections are viral, without a throat culture it is impossible to distinguish a viral infection of the throat from the bacterial infection of strep throat. After appropriate cultures have been obtained and a strep throat is diagnosed, you should take the appropriate antibiotic for a full ten days. Failure to do so puts you at risk for a very uncommon complication these days, that of acute rheumatic fever. It is especially important for patients who have had acute rheumatic fever, or who have a strong family history of acute rheumatic fever, to get prompt diagnosis and treatment of strep throat. When the bacteria causing a strep throat (the Streptococcus) is not promptly killed, it elicits a strong antibody response from the patient's immune system. This antibody response attacks not only the Streptococcus but also certain tissues of the body including heart valves, sometimes permanently damaging them. Rheumatic heart disease is the result.

Pneumonia

About half of all pneumonias in adults are caused by bacteria (the other half by viruses). Such bacterial pneumonias may occur out of the blue in a previously healthy individual. The symptoms include fever and chills and a cough producing infected phlegm. There may be pain on one side of the chest, a pain made worse by deep breathing or coughing, so-called pleuritic chest pain or pleurisy. In young healthy adults suffering from a simple pneumonia, treatment may be entirely appropriate with antibiotics taken by mouth in an outpatient setting. For people with chronic bronchitis and emphysema (usually from cigarette smoking), pneumonias are usually treated in-hospital with intravenous antibiotics.

Not infrequently, young adults may suffer from a mild persistent pneumonia, now called **primary atypical pneumonia** but in former days often referred to as "walking" pneumonia. The symptoms of this pneumonia are slightly different: The cough is bothersome, and especially so at night. Fever may be mild, and the cough rarely produces an infected sputum. There may be an associated earache. Pleurisy, pain on breathing, is not common. Specific diagnosis is important because the organism causing "walking" pneumonia, Mycoplasma, is *not* sensitive to the penicillins. Because the pneumonia occurs in healthy young adults, almost always it can be treated in the outpatient setting with oral antibiotics. Both erythromycin and tetracycline are effective antibiotics for this type of pneumonia.

There are many other, less common infectious diseases which space does not allow us to discuss here. Although we cannot examine them specifically, remembering the difference between bacteria and virus, and antibiotic use versus host defenses (to be discussed below) is very helpful in understanding diagnosis and treatment of infectious disease. But before we examine host defenses and the body's immune system, let's examine a case report to illustrate another aspect of bacterial infection.

Ptomaine Poisoning

During the final year of medical school, the prospective new intern interviews at various hospitals of his or her choice. The procedure is very much like that of college admissions. One such candidate journeyed to our hospital for an interview. The evening before his interview, on the way to the hospital, he stopped at an interstate fast-food restaurant and ordered the tuna salad. Two hours later he was in our emergency room with severe vomiting, abdominal cramps, and profuse diarrhea. He had become dehydrated and required intravenous therapy. As interns ourselves, we had a great deal of sympathy for his predicament. He had an interview in the morning. We rehydrated him with infusion of intravenous solutions, saw that he got his rest, dusted him off, spruced him up, and called our chief in the morning to come to the bedside for his admission interview. We suggested that the chief be easy on our patient. The interview went well. The chief gave him a job.

What happened to the student was this: He had eaten tuna salad contaminated with a bacterium called Staphylococcus. The bacterium had not multiplied to the extent to decompose the tuna salad (and so become easily detected), but there was enough Staphylococcus in the salad to cause his food poisoning. It was not the bacterium per se that produced the symptoms but rather a toxic by-product produced by the bacterium, a so-called toxin, that gave rise to the student's illness. Proper refrigeration of food prevents the formation of the toxin. Once it is formed, however, the toxin is remarkably resistant to heating and will not be destroyed by cooking.

HOST DEFENSES: THE IMMUNE SYSTEM

Let's return to the palace metaphor again. When we consider the threat of infectious disease, we are concerned with a threat from outside the palace, rather than threat of destruction from within as is the case with cancer. Accordingly, an invader may slip in through an open window, a crack in the foundation, or a door left slightly ajar. Once having gained entrance through a chink in the palace's external armor, contending with the invader becomes the responsibility of the palace guard. With respect to the human body, the skin, microscopic hairs and mucous in the respiratory tract, the cough reflex, and even acid in the stomach are the initial armor to external threat. The palace guard is an even more complicated internal barrier than this, consisting of many kinds of white blood cells together with their special weapon, **antibodies.**

Antibodies

Antibodies are small molecules of protein manufactured on-the-spot to attack a specific invading microbe. They are made in response to invasion by an infective agent. Should the infecting agent constitute a threat on a second occasion, the body "remembers" how to make the antibody more quickly, more efficiently, and in greater amounts. This is the whole basis for immunization. *Antibodies perform a great many roles.* For instance, they may neutralize the poisons or toxins produced by certain bacteria, such as the toxin which was produced in our case of ptomaine poisoning discussed above. Antibodies may neutralize viruses themselves or cause bacteria to clump together, thereby rendering them less mobile and a more ready target for destruction by white blood cells. Antibodies can cause other white corpuscles to release their chemical weapons in response to infection, and they may, as in the case of the common cold, prevent viruses from adhering to and infecting certain tissues. If a cell becomes infected with a virus, antibodies attached to that cell may coordinate chemical reactions to destroy the viruses contained within.

White Blood Cell Immunity

Special white blood cells have a central role in the immune response — they may be thought of as the generals of the palace guard. Other white blood cells, the foot soldiers of the palace guard, attack and destroy bacteria. A third class, the artillery, manufacture both antibodies and other chemicals to cause destruction of foreign infectious agents. The generals of the palace guard are called the T-4 lymphocytes. In response to infection, they become very busy with a great many things. T-4 lymphocytes, for example, release chemicals in response to infection, chemicals to stimulate the bone marrow to make more foot soldiers to fight the infection. The T-4 lymphocytes, the generals, cause other white blood cells to manufacture chemicals to kill virus particles and stop the reproduction of viruses. (These chemicals are called **interferons.**) It is not difficult to understand that when a disease attacks the palace guard itself, the integrity of the palace will be very greatly threatened. This is so with AIDS, a virus which attacks the palace guard generals, the T-4 lymphocytes, themselves. We will discuss AIDS a bit later.

VIRUSES

Viruses are among the simplest of living organisms. They consist only of a bit of chromosome, or genetic, material, contained in an envelope of protein. They contain nothing more. They invade a cell and trick the cell's chromosome material into making more virus. There are more than 400 viruses which infect humans. Because viruses are unaffected by antibiotics, immunization must be relied upon to prevent, and host defenses relied on to fight, virus infection. Viruses are the cause of such widely dissimilar diseases as warts and smallpox, hepatitis and diarrhea, poliomyelitis and influenza, rabies and yellow fever. We cannot examine all of these viral infections in detail but an understanding of one or two will give you the appreciation of the magnitude of the problem of viral infection and the methods by which we presently cope with viruses.

Influenza

There is great misunderstanding about just what *is* influenza. Many viral upper respiratory infections are termed "the flu" by both patient and doctor. Anything from a runny nose, a bout of diarrhea, a week or more of dry cough and malaise, abdominal cramps, and fever are mistakenly called "the flu." True influenza is an unforgettable illness. High fever, shaking chills, severe headache, severe muscle aching, and a feeling of extreme prostration render the patient bedridden for a week or more. Other viral upper respiratory infections may cause a runny nose and sinus congestion but influenza more characteristically features a very dry nose and throat and a dry cough. There is the typical central chest pain aggravated by the dry hacking cough. Without a complicating pneumonia, the fever of influenza may be gone in three to four days and the illness is over within about a week.

Influenza is caused by one particular virus, a virus having many types and designations, which have given rise to a confusing array of names: Asian flu, Hong Kong flu, Russian flu, swine flu, and others. Consider this analogy: Just as dogs may be setters, poodles, or hounds, influenza viruses come in three types, A, B, and C. Within each of these types of influenza virus, there are a number of subtypes caused by chemical variations within the virus particle itself. These subtypes are designated A1, A2, etc., as in English and Irish setters. These subtypes are named for a place of origin. For example, influenza A/Texas 77 originated in Texas in 1977. Each subtype is itself subject to variations, just as two Irish setters never look exactly alike. These variations within a subtype produce differences sufficient enough to prevent any antibody response from "remembering" a previous influenza infection. Past influenza infection thus may not afford immunity against the next epidemic. An influenza immunization attempts to trick the body's host defenses into thinking that influenza has infected the body, causing the body's defenses to produce antibodies to one or more of the influenza subtypes. In this way, if the real thing comes along, the antibody-manufacturing system "remembers" and quickly springs into action.

Epidemics of A-type virus occur in cycles of about every two to four years, whereas influenza B epidemics cycle every four to six years. Very rarely does a worldwide epidemic or so-called **pandemic** occur. There have been three pandemics in this century. In 1917-18, 500 million people contracted influenza and 20 million people died during three waves of a pandemic caused by an influenza A-subtype which was known also to infect pigs. Not all the people who died in that pandemic of 1917-18 were old and debilitated; one of every sixty-seven army soldiers with influenza died of it. When the A-swine subtype which caused this 1917-18 pandemic was found in 1975 in five army recruits with influenza at Fort Dix, the very real possibility of another swine-flu pandemic prompted the mass immunization program of 1976-77.

The 1957 Asian influenza pandemic, which was also caused by an A-subtype virus, spread like wildfire, the result in part of an international congress of high school students held in Iowa and attended by 1800 students from forty-three states as well as countries abroad. The attack rate of this pandemic was incredible. I remember going to school on a Monday in 1957 to find only a substitute teacher, the town bully, and the meanest girl in the ninth grade. It was a very dark day indeed. The mortality with the 1957 pandemic was far less than with the earlier 1917 pandemic but not because of anything modern medicine could do. This influenza virus subtype merely produced a less lethal illness.

There is still no cure for influenza. The drug *amantadine* may attenuate or shorten the course of some influenza-A infections if the drug is started early enough in the disease, but it does not cure the disease. The illness must run its course and the body depends upon its own host defenses for ultimate eradication of the virus. Aspirin, fluids, and bedrest help the symptoms. Codeine relieves the dry cough and the chest pain.

Remember: Antibiotics are of no use and may indeed be harmful by promoting growth of highly virulent bacteria within the lungs already compromised and weakened by viral infection.

A persistent fever after three or four days, a cough which becomes productive of infected phlegm, marked prostration, and a wet rattling chest, signal the development of a complicating pneumonia, which can be extremely dangerous. You should notify your doctor immediately if these symptoms occur.

You can increase your chances of avoiding an influenza infection by getting an influenza immunization. Although it is impossible to be vaccinated against all of the various types and subtypes of influenza virus, it *is* possible to make an educated guess about which types may be about to descend upon us. The educated guess comes about in this way: One considers the cyclical nature of epidemics. One keeps in mind the most recently isolated influenza subtypes. The virus which caused Hong Kong flu in 1972 — a B-type virus — was manifested again in 1978-79. A-type Brazil and A-type USSR viruses are so similar that vaccination against one will afford protection against both viruses. Usually flu shots contain killed virus from three distinct strains, usually two A-strains and a B-strain. The B-strain will be that subtype most likely to be coming around again in its four to six year cycle. Seventy percent of those vaccinated obtain immunity to these and similar influenza virus strains for a period of three to six months.

Many people commonly believe that flu shots afford protection against other virus infections. This is not so. Patients continually tell me that they have gotten a flu shot and "haven't had a cold in a year." This may be because of good host defenses, or luck, or both, but it is not because of the flu shot. Alternatively, a flu shot will not "cause" the flu or a flu-like illness although with a small minority of patients, five percent or so, there may be a mild, fever-like reaction to the shot. This reaction with fever, muscle aches, and fatigue lasts only one to two days and is mild. About one third of those vaccinated get swelling and tenderness at the site of the injection. If you are allergic to eggs or egg protein, you should *not* have a flu shot.

Who Should Get a Flu Shot?

The following people should strongly consider getting a flu shot every year:

- Those who are at high risk of dying from epidemic influenza, including anyone over sixty-five years of age
- Those of any age with heart disease
- Those people having chronic diseases
- Pregnant women with the above
- For all others, especially those with a high risk of exposure, such as teachers and medical personnel, and those providing essential community services, the benefits and risks of immunizations against influenza have to be considered by both patient and doctor.

The Common Cold

Why is it so easy to immunize against influenza, and so effective to prevent poliomyelitis through immunization, and yet so impossible to prevent the common cold? One reason for this is the extreme variability of viruses causing the common cold and the lack of predictable cycling of virus epidemics as we have experienced with influenza. Many types of viruses are known to cause the common cold. Rhinoviruses and coronaviruses probably account for about fifty percent of infections we call "the common cold." But another thirty to fifty percent of such infections, although presumed to be viral, have never had an identifiable agent associated with the infection. And even rhinoviruses have over one hundred subtypes. Antibodies to a particular subtype of rhinovirus *do* lessen an infection with that subtype. However, *this* antibody may not totally prevent infection with *that* subtype of rhinovirus. This is probably because most of the infection occurs in the mucous membranes of the nose and sinuses, areas that the antibodies have a difficult time getting to in order to fight the virus.

The old adage, "a cold will last seven days with treatment, and a week without," is still true. There is no specific treatment for the common cold. Antibiotics are of no value. The use of vitamin C is debatable. Some evidence does indicate that the taking of vitamin C during a respiratory illness like the common cold *may* shorten the duration of the illness.

Immunization Against Infectious Diseases

Effective immunization exists for certain bacterial and viral infections. Immunization entails the injection of microbes (bacteria and viruses) or parts of microbes, either in live but ineffective form or in killed form. The body's immune system "sees" the infective agent and mounts an antibody response to that agent. Should a bonafide infection come along, the body's defenses are ready for it. Table 12-1 gives immunization schedules for both children and adults.

TABLE 12-1 Immunization Schedules

Children	
Time	*Shots*
At two months of age	Diphtheria, pertusis, tetanus (DPT), oral polio vaccine
At four months	DPT, oral polio vaccine
At six months	DPT
At fifteen months	Measles, mumps, and rubella
At eighteen months	DPT, polio
At twenty-four months	Hemophilus B vaccine
At five-six years	DPT, polio
At fifteen years	Diphtheria, tetanus (and every ten years thereafter)

(continues)

TABLE 12–1   continued

Adults (18 years and older)	
Shots	*Indications*
Influenza vaccine	Adults at high risk and high exposure (see text)
Pneumovax (pneumococcal vaccine)	Adults at high risk of pneumonia, especially those with chronic lung disease and the elderly
Hepatitis B vaccine	Adults at risk of occupational, environmental, or social exposure to hepatitis B virus
Diphtheria, tetanus	All adults every ten years
Measles vaccine	Adults (born after 1956) who have not been vaccinated against measles or who have not had documented infection with measles
German measles vaccine (rubella)	Adults who have not been previously vaccinated against rubella or who have not had documented infection with rubella

AIDS: ACQUIRED IMMUNODEFICIENCY SYNDROME

Why is it that one viral disease, smallpox, has been eradicated from the face of the earth and yet the AIDS virus so far seems impossible to control? How can it be that the oral polio vaccine confers complete immunity against the poliomyelitis virus and yet such a vaccine has not yet been developed for the AIDS virus?

Certain white corpuscles, the **lymphocytes,** play an integral role in the body's own defense mechanisms, as we have discussed above. Among these lymphocytes, the T-4 lymphocyte, or helper T-cell, plays a central role in directing the body's immune response. It may be thought of as the general of the palace guard. These T-4 lymphocytes recognize a foreign invader and help set into motion immune responses from other white corpuscles, which in turn produce antibodies to fight an infection. T-4 lymphocytes also direct other lymphocytes (T-8 lymphocytes) to kill cells infected by virus. Other white blood cells, the monocytes and macrophages, are also under direct control of T-4 cells during an infection. Hence, when the human body is infected with bacteria, the T-4 lymphocyte controls the production of antibody by other lymphocytes to fight that bacteria. The T-4 lymphocyte directs other lymphocytes to attack the bacteria. And finally, the T-4 lymphocyte, in many other complicated ways, directs a well-orchestrated immune response against the invading bacteria.

The essence of the AIDS dilemma is this: The AIDS virus infects and destroys the T-4 lymphocyte. The palace guard's general is lost. The central control of the immune response is itself destroyed by the viral infection. Hence, in the late stages of AIDS, the person infected with the AIDS virus is unable to fight off common, minor infections from yeast (Candida), herpes simplex virus, cytomegalovirus (a common infection producing mild disease in healthy people), and Pneumocystis carinii pneumonia (a very rare pneumonia seen *only* in patients with lowered resistance). Simply stated, this is how AIDS patients die: The T-4 lymphocyte system is destroyed, the body's defense mechanisms are rendered useless, and the patient is attacked and killed by microbes, which in the healthy patient are of only minor concern.

Paradoxically, patients infected with the AIDS virus mount an impressive antibody response against the virus. But this seems to make no difference in the course of the disease. In our present knowledge of research, it seems that conventional immunization exciting an antibody response to the various parts of the virus is of no help to the patient. Present research focuses upon a particular protein on the surface of the T-4 lymphocyte, the protein called CD-4 antigen, to which the virus attaches before it destroys the T-4 lymphocyte. If, through immunization, antibodies can be developed to block the binding of the virus to the CD-4 antigen on the surface of the T-4 lymphocyte, perhaps an effective vaccine can be developed. The development of a vaccine against AIDS is also thwarted because the virus can hide inside cells, can change the nature of its protein coating and therefore "hide" from an antibody response, and because the AIDS virus can insert its own genetic material within the chromosomes of its host cell, with a very long latency period before reproducing itself.

Because the AIDS virus is transmitted from one individual to the other by infected semen or vaginal fluid during intercourse or by direct transfer of blood containing the AIDS virus into the bloodstream of another, infection is *not* a casual occurrence. AIDS is *not* the highly contagious viral infection that we see with measles, for example, or with influenza. Trauma from sexual intercourse, especially through anal intercourse, and intravenous drug use from shared, infected syringes are the most common methods of infection. At greatest risk, therefore, are gay or bisexual men, followed thereafter by intravenous drug users. Because of promiscuity, and probably because of their high rate of intravenous drug use, prostitutes are also at high risk of having infection. People who are strictly heterosexual are at much lower risk, although promiscuity increases the risk, particularly in areas where intravenous drug use is common. When considering AIDS, the following points are very important to keep in mind:

- Promiscuity places one at greatly increased risk.
- Sex without a condom with a person infected by the AIDS virus is dangerous.
- The use of condoms greatly reduces the risk of contracting AIDS.
- Sharing drug needles with an infected person is most likely to be *lethal*.
- AIDS is a universal problem and not likely soon to be solved.
- A patient may be infected with the AIDS virus for eight years or longer before ever becoming ill and, therefore, outwardly manifesting the disease.
- The HIV blood test may not become positive until six months from the time of exposure to the virus.

- There is *no* evidence that transmission of the virus occurs through mosquito bites.
- *Casual* contact (handshake, touching, hugging, etc.) will not transmit the virus from one infected individual to another.
- There is no evidence that sharing food or utensils with an infected person will transmit the disease.

CONCLUSION

Infectious diseases comprise a whole array of potential invaders to the human body. Antibiotics are only one of many ways to fight infection, and they are not always the most appropriate treatment. An informed patient needs to understand the nature of infectious disease, how to prevent needless infection, whether from AIDS or measles, and when to recognize signs of worsening infection. This chapter is not meant to be and is not an exhaustive discussion of infectious diseases. It is meant to give you a frame of reference from which to discuss problems of infectious disease with your physician.

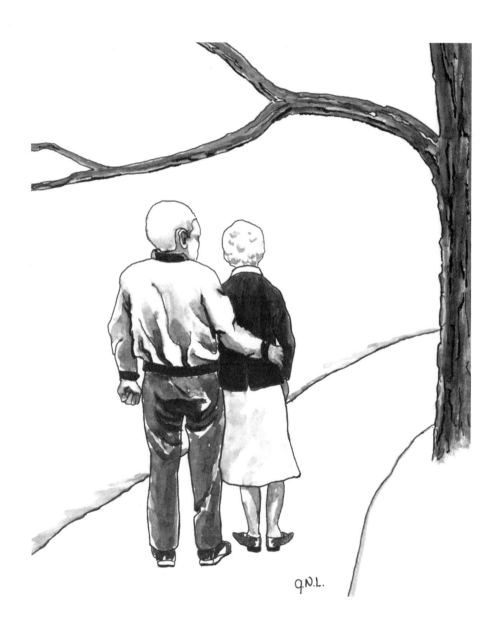

13

Problems of Sexuality

"The omnipresent process of sex, as it is woven into the whole texture of our man's or woman's body, is the pattern of all the process of our life."

Havelock Ellis

Not infrequently, sexual problems require the help of a physician. Four problem areas most commonly confronting the primary physician are:

- Sex education, or rather the lack of it
- Sexually transmitted diseases
- Impotence and decreased sex drive
- The use of contraception

Let's address the most vital concern first.

THE PROBLEM OF SEX EDUCATION

What accounts for the high rate of teenage pregnancy? Many argue that liberalized sexual attitudes are to blame, or socioeconomic factors are the problem, or family discord, or rampant promiscuity. Well, perhaps a few girls really do get pregnant to seek revenge upon their parents. *But eight out of ten girls between the ages of ten and nineteen who become pregnant really did not wish to become pregnant.* Few of these girls use any contraception at all. They are neither promiscuous nor vindictive. They are quite simply misinformed; they lack any comprehensive education in sexuality, an education which is most certainly their right, and which we as parents owe to them.

There are prevalent myths about sexuality, myths leading to irresponsible behavior. Let's examine some of these.

Sexual Myth #1. It is commonly believed that sex education itself — that open discussion about sex — leads to experimentation, to promiscuity, and to an increase in teenage pregnancy. This is a belief not held by teenagers, certainly, but rather by many parents, clergy, and teachers who are most able to promote sex education. Medical research has clearly shown that sex education leads to *more* responsible behavior rather than *less,* and it promotes postponement of sexual intercourse among teenagers rather than encouraging promiscuity. Those teenagers given sex education in the schools and in the home are more apt to act with understanding and caution. Those without sex education simply take risks.

Sexual Myth #2. This myth goes something like this: "If you *plan* to have sex, that is immoral. Spontaneous sex is acceptable morally because one cannot help oneself and is not responsible for one's actions." A loaded pistol! Here is a myth we can all understand. Briefly stated, the more spontaneity in sexual matters and the less planning involved, the less sinful one is.

The psychological conflict here is complex. The teenager denies that any planning of sexual behavior occurs. This denial is most common among those young people most guilty about their sexuality. In the extreme case, intense denial on the part of a teenage girl may include denial that coitus ever actually occurred. Whether the girl feels simply out of control of the situation, and thus not morally responsible, or whether she denies that coitus ever occurred (when indeed it did!), an unwanted pregnancy is often the result. When a teenager holds that only spontaneous sex is moral, or at least not immoral, such a teenager trades responsible behavior for passion. How ironic that those young people who are made to feel most guilty about their sexuality tend also not to use any contraception, since that would involve planning! They tend also *not* to refrain from sexual intercourse during the teenage years. Open discussions about sexuality with teenagers would allow them to think about their sexuality and permit them to behave responsibly, rather than forcing them simply to feel guilty.

Sexual Myth #3. Most teenagers believe that all of their peers are having sexual intercourse. In subscribing to this myth, they believe that they are missing out on something, or perhaps they are in some way abnormal. Each thinks that he or she is the only virgin in town. The sexual revolution among teenagers has been grossly exaggerated. It is *promiscuity* among teenagers that is the *real* myth.

Still, the media would have us think otherwise, that teenage promiscuity is the norm. This leads many teenagers to believe that they are being left out. This belief in turn leads to irresponsible, unplanned behavior. If young people can be made to see that *not* everyone is 'doing it' and if we can support our teenagers' right to say "no," we can begin to dispell this myth.

Sexual Myth #4. There is much confusion these days about sex and love. This is nothing new. The issue has been confused for some 4,000 years now. Young women *especially* believe that sex and love are equated; that is, that sex means love. Teenage girls have believed since antiquity that if they have sex with someone, he will be more likely to love them afterwards. By discussing with young people the difference between love and sexual attraction, by examining openly the very common intense physical reaction that occurs in the teenage years, we can begin to help teenagers separate out these feelings and begin to act responsibly.

Sexual Myth #5. Prevalent among teenage boys is the belief that "no" means "yes." Teenage girls compound the problem by believing that it is okay for a boy to force a girl to have sex if she has "turned him on." When these two beliefs meet head-on, the result is almost always a teenage pregnancy.

One person says "no" and means it, but may give in to another's further advances. We need to discuss with our teenagers how to say "no," how to be blunt, and how to dampen the ardor of the aggressive partner. When was the last time you discussed such topics with your teenagers?

Sexual Myth #6. There is considerable misinformation about the menstrual cycle in relation to when pregnancy can occur in the cycle. It is commonly believed that one can *never* get pregnant during menstruation, that therefore sexual intercourse during a girl's period is absolutely safe. *This is not true.* A woman can get pregnant through sexual intercourse on any day of her menstrual cycle, menstrual days included. The reasons *why* this may occur involve a discussion of ovulation, the viability of sperm and ovum, and where fertilization actually takes place — topics of human sexuality which may occupy one or two hours of a sex education course in school.

In a large survey of teenagers, less than half of those surveyed knew the most likely time during a woman's menstrual cycle when pregnancy *may* occur, and less than half knew that a woman can get pregnant even if her sexual partner withdraws before ejaculation takes place. Many girls believe also that they are too young to get pregnant, or don't have sex frequently enough to get pregnant, or can't get pregnant because they are standing up during intercourse, or because they didn't have an orgasm during coitus. Girls who have sexual intercourse infrequently and do not get pregnant may actually believe that it can *never* happen to them.

Sexual Myth #7. Teenage boys commonly believe that condoms reduce sexual pleasure; therefore they do not use them. In truth, condoms reduce pleasure only when they are allowed to interrupt lovemaking. One does not have to hide oneself in a closet while putting on a condom — using a condom can be a part of the sexual experience itself. It does not necessarily reduce pleasure. It is responsible behavior.

Sexual Myth #8. For most teenagers, sex means sexual intercourse. There is very little discussion with and among teenagers about noncoital forms of sexual behavior; that is, sexual behavior other than intercourse. Yet lovemaking also means holding, cuddling, touching, mutual masturbation, as well as sexual intercourse. Young people who are allowed to discuss these behaviors openly and examine them can make distinctions in the kinds of relationships and experiences they want. Not all relationships have to be sexual, and not all sexual relationships have to include sexual intercourse.

The Question Box   Whether we like it or not, every teenager will be faced with decisions about having sexual intercourse: with whom, under what circumstances, and with or without contraception. If we choose to "shield" our young people from information on human sexuality, experience has shown that we are merely pushing them toward irresponsible behavior. If it is true that eight out of ten girls who get pregnant during the teenage years *did not wish to become pregnant,* then as adults withholding sex education from them *we* become very much a part of the problem.

Some years ago, I had an opportunity to teach a course in human sexuality at a Catholic college for women. There were approximately 250 students in the course, predominantly students in their senior year. The college was one with very high academic standards and with orthodox Christian beliefs. Because of the nature of the course content itself, questions during class were often embarrassing for the students to ask. I began a practice of soliciting from them anonymous questions, which they would place in a question box kept at the front of the lecture hall. I reviewed their questions and answered them at the beginning of the next lecture. The question box was always stuffed.

What follows is a list of some of the questions those students asked. As you read through them, ask yourself whether these are concerns representative of those of most young adults? Ask yourself whether these questions deserve an answer? Are these prospective mothers well informed? Are these women immoral? Do they have no values? Do they have no right to sex education? Here are their questions:

- Are there any drugs that affect birth control pills? (Ans: For all practical purposes there are none.)
- You stated in class that sex seems to be a problem in two-thirds of marriages. Can you tell me where a man or a woman can go for help in this matter if they don't have a family doctor or if they don't feel

that the family doctor is the right person to see?
(Ans: Find a well-qualified psychologist or psychiatrist, using the approach outlined in Chapter Two.)

- Is there really a distinction, as stated in the textbook, between a vaginal and a clitoral orgasm?
(Ans: There is no distinction. Some orgasms are more enjoyable than others, just as some sunsets are more beautiful than others.)

- Is there any relationship between the pill and anemia?
(Ans: Birth control pills do not cause an anemia.)

- If a woman has intercourse the day before her period starts and the egg is fertilized, will her period start the next day or is everything stopped the minute she becomes pregnant?
(Ans: Most likely, menstruation will start and the egg will not implant within the uterus; the woman will not become pregnant.)

- What is oral intercourse? Is it common? Is it normal?
(Ans: It is oral-genital kissing. It is common and normal.)

- Would one be able to continue taking tranquilizers daily for their nine months' pregnancy and give birth to a normal child?
(Ans: *Any* drug, with the exception of aspirin and probably penicillin, can cause birth defects, especially in the first three months of pregnancy. If the tranquilizers are absolutely essential during the pregnancy, the woman should be switched to that tranquilizer *least* likely to cause birth defects, under direction of a physician.)

- What percentage of women who are on the pill develop blood clots? Must they necessarily have had a case of phlebitis or other blood disorder in the family to have this occur?
(Ans: The incidence of blood clots on the pill is extremely small, but more common in women who

have had phlebitis before, or whose family members are prone to blood clots.)

- If it is known that one has a tipped uterus, is it harder to get pregnant?
  (Ans: *Occasionally* it is more difficult to get pregnant with a tipped uterus, but there are simple positional techniques the woman can be taught to enhance pregnancy.)

- What causes menstrual cramps? One misunderstanding: The diameter of the cervix limits the flow and the pressure of the remaining menses in the cervix causes pain. Is this true?
  (Ans: Menstrual cramps are caused by contractions of the muscles of the uterus. There is no relationship of menstrual pain to the diameter of the cervix limiting flow.)

- Do marijuana and hallucinogens affect birth control pills so they aren't as effective?
  (Ans: Only if, because of the drug high, the birth control pill is not taken as prescribed. But some hallucinogens *may* cause chromosomal problems and birth defects.)

- What are the chances of a person who is a voyeur or exhibitionist becoming a normal functioning person? Can a marriage to a person with either of these problems be sexually successful?
  (Ans: Both voyeurism and exhibitionism, so-called sexual "perversions," are eminently treatable by psychiatrists and, with successful treatment, marriage to such a person can be sexually successful.)

- Is oral-genital sex physically unhealthy for a couple?
  (Ans: No, it is not.)

- Isn't an ideal relationship when both achieve orgasm together? Everything you read states this.
  (Ans: Simultaneous orgasm is enjoyable, but not the ideal. It is often more pleasurable for couples when one focuses on the orgasm of the other and then vice versa.)

- Does oral sex contribute to urinary infections in the female?

(Ans: If the male partner has "cold sores" in the mouth, herpes simplex infections, that viral infection may be transmitted to the woman's labia. Although not strictly a urinary infection, it is a genital infection caused by oral sex.)

- Is it painful if during intercourse the penis thrusts up against the cervix?
  (Ans: It is not normally painful, unless there exists an infection of the cervix or uterus.)
- How often should a person who has intercourse regularly douche? Doesn't all that semen and vaginal sweat cause odor? Also, what happens to the semen after intercourse? Where does it go?
  (Ans: Regular douching is not necessary. No odor is caused. The body cleanses itself. Regular douching in fact may make a woman prone to vaginal infections.)
- Can too much masturbation serve to overstimulate or numb the genitals and desensitize other areas?
  (Ans: No. Absolutely not.)
- When a man has sex with a virgin, is it possible for him to break her hymen with a prophylactic on and still have the prophylactic effective as a birth control measure, so he can safely continue having intercourse with her?
  (Ans: It is not only possible, it is probable. Only very rarely would a prophylactic, or condom, break under such circumstances.)
- Are there other birth control measures a virgin can use besides taking the pill?
  (Ans: Yes there are, but they are not as successful in preventing pregnancy. See the contraception section of this chapter.)
- How long after coitus does a girl have to wait to be able to detect pregnancy in her urine, assuming she became pregnant at the time of coitus?
  (Ans: Four weeks after conception.)
- Is there any possible danger to developing sexual organs if you take the pill before twenty-one?
  (Ans: No danger.)
- I am no longer afraid of getting married.

(Ans: Then, this course in sex education has been a success.)

SEXUALLY TRANS-MITTED DISEASES

A second common problem in human sexuality is that of sexually transmitted diseases. We have already considered the most serious, most catastrophic, of those illnesses, Acquired Immune Deficiency Syndrome, or AIDS, in Chapter Twelve. Here we shall consider the more common, and far less serious, infections transmitted through sexual intercourse.

Herpes Simplex.   Herpes infection is the most common of the sexually transmitted diseases. It is caused by a virus, the herpes simplex virus, which produces small blisters or shallow ulcers on the glans of the penis or on the penile shaft and, in the woman, most commonly on the labia and around the clitoris. These lesions are usually painful and, with first infection, can be severely so. I will never forget admitting to the hospital a young woman, a high school sophomore, who ultimately proved to have a first infection with herpes simplex virus. She had a temperature of 103 degrees Fahrenheit, shaking chills, and intense inflammation and swelling of the labia and vaginal tissues. Within a week all symptoms resolved.

Herpes infection usually lasts for about a week, during which time sexual activity should be stopped, both because of pain and because of the possibility of transmitting the disease. An oral and topical antiviral agent, acyclovir, can shorten the *duration* of the initial infection and lessen the severity of frequent recurrences, which often happen with herpes infection. Acyclovir, however, does not offer cure.

Venereal Warts.   Also caused by a virus, and also quite common, venereal warts are painless, small, wart-like growths occurring on the penis, vulva, perineum, and anus. The warts contain virus and are infective, which means they can be spread to sexual partners and will also spread locally from the initial point of infection.

There are many forms of treatment; all are successful. A topical solution of podophyllin can be applied; this treatment, however, tends to be irritating and sometimes quite painful. Alternatively, freezing the warts with liquid nitrogen or using laser surgery can remove the warts. It should be obvious that the sexual partner of a patient with venereal warts should also be observed for the appearance of such warts which should be treated promptly if they occur.

Candidiasis. Candidiasis or moniliasis is a very common vaginal infection. It is caused by a fungus normally present in the vagina. It is not strictly transmitted through sexual intercourse, although sexual transmission can occur. Male sexual partners tend to be asymptomatic carriers of the fungus, reinfecting the woman unless they are also treated.

Candidiasis, "the yeast infection," produces vaginal burning and itching and a thick vaginal discharge, cottage cheese-like in character. Intercourse is usually painful during this infection.

There are many conditions which predispose a woman to infection with the yeast Candida, including treatment with antibiotics for a urinary tract infection, treatment with cortisone-like preparations, or use of birth control pills. Candidiasis tends to be more frequent in pregnant women and in those who have diabetes mellitus.

Treatment is usually very effective with topical antifungal agents. Remember, however, to have your sexual partner treated as well, if you have one.

A college coed came to me after several weeks of suffering from a yeast infection. She had endured intense burning and itching of the vaginal tissues together with a profuse discharge characteristic of yeast infection, putting up with it for so long because of fear of moral judgment. Though she was a virgin, she was convinced that somehow she had contracted a venereal disease. She had not. There are two lessons here. Both bear repeating again and again:

- No disease confers with it a moral judgment.

- The most common infections of the vagina are *not* necessarily transmitted through sexual intercourse.

Trichomoniasis. Trichomoniasis is caused by a small, one-celled animal, a protozoan, which is neither a bacterium nor a virus. (An amoeba, for example, is a protozoan). The infection *may* be spread through sexual intercourse, but not necessarily. The cysts of Trichomonas may normally be found in the vagina. Virgins may certainly contract trichomoniasis when excessive growth of the organisms occurs. The infection, usually symptomatic in the woman and asymptomatic in the man, causes an intense malodorous vaginal discharge, usually with vaginal burning and pain on intercourse. There is less itching than with candidiasis. Diagnosis depends upon microscopic analysis of the vaginal discharge by a physician and treatment both of the symptomatic woman and the asymptomatic sexual partner, if there is one. Treatment is very successful with the use of metronidazole (Flagyl).

The fact that a woman may contract trichomoniasis *without* having had any sexual encounter with a man also so infected can cause problems. I had a patient with typical trichomoniasis for whom I prescribed treatment. I explained to her how the disease may occur devoid of any sexual exposure to the organism — that the organism may occur *normally* in the vagina but simply get out of hand. I told her also that her husband should be treated since he may have become infected through intercouse with her and be carrying the organism. He could then reinfect her or become symptomatic from the infection himself. I gave her a prescription for her husband. He stormed into the office, convinced that she had been unfaithful. Only after an exhaustive discussion, and reference to many medical textbooks, could he be reassured.

Gonorrhea. Herpes simplex virus, candidiasis, and trichomoniasis are more commonly symptomatic in women and asymptomatic in men. Gonorrheal infection more commonly produces symptoms in men and is asymptomatic in women. In the male patient with gonorrhea, an intense, painful penile discharge literally *drives* the patient to medical attention. Treatment of the male with appropriate antibiotic therapy is highly successful. In the woman, gonorrheal infection is quite common, particularly in those who have multiple sexual partners. Infected women may have no symptoms; the infection is usually diagnosed in these women when gonorrheal infection in their male partners becomes manifest.

Gonorrhea in the woman may produce vaginal discharge with itching, pain on intercourse, burning upon urination, lower abdominal pain, and, with advancing infection, fever, nausea, and increased abdominal pain. Effective antibiotic therapy is available.

Chlamydia.   Infection with Chlamydia is more common than with gonorrhea. Like trichomoniasis and candidiasis, Chlamydia infection does not have to occur through sexual intercourse, although those women with multiple sexual partners are more likely to be infected. The infection produces lower abdominal pain and a slightly increased vaginal discharge or scant penile discharge in the male. There is usually burning on urination, but rarely fever. Diagnosis of Chlamydia infection is simple, but *special* tests for the infection must be done. The organism is *not* sensitive to penicillin as is the gonococcus causing gonorrhea. Chlamydia is sensitive to tetracycline or doxycycline, both very safe antibiotics except in pregnant women, who should be treated with sulfonamides.

Syphilis.   Syphilis has become quite an uncommon disease. In its initial stages it is characterized by a painless shallow-based ulcer at the point of sexual contact, wherever that may be. Remember, the ulcer of herpes simplex is *painful;* that of syphilis is *painless.* The ulcer of syphilis never blisters, whereas that of herpes always blisters initially. Syphilis usually has only *one* ulcer in the majority of cases, whereas herpes simplex infection produces *many* ulcers in groups. If the lymph glands in the groin are swollen because of infection from syphilis, they will be painless and nontender whereas in herpes infection they will be painful and tender.

If syphilis is not diagnosed in its initial or *primary* stage, most patients will later develop a *secondary* phase weeks or months after the initial contact. This stage, secondary syphilis, features a body rash most typically involving the palms and soles as well as the trunk. The rash is usually not itchy. Constitutional symptoms such as fever, fatigue, weight loss, and headache are quite common. Blood tests for syphilis are always positive at this stage whereas in other rashes, with which syphilis may be confused (rashes caused by drugs for example), the test for syphilis will be negative. Treatment is still very effective with penicillin.

IMPOTENCE AND DECREASED SEX DRIVE

In discussing sexual dysfunction it is important to remember some very important distinctions. Most sexual dysfunction occurs because of *psychological* reasons rather than *physical* reasons. That is the first distinction. Physicians refer to this as **psychogenic** (psychological) versus **organic** (physical) cause. The second distinction addresses the *type* of sexual dysfunction. One may have a normal *desire* for sex (libido) and yet find an inhibition of sexual excitement or an *inability to perform* (loss of potency). Alternatively, sexual dysfunction may occur because of loss of desire altogether; in this instance ability to perform or degree of sexual excitement cannot be an issue.

An exhaustive discussion of sexual dysfunction is beyond the scope of this book, just as is comprehensive treatment of sexual dysfunction beyond the scope of any primary care physician. Still, with sexual problems that is a good place to start, in a doctor's office discussing your problems with a physician whom you trust. Regrettably, such discussions seldom happen. Physicians almost never take a sexual history from their patients. It either does not occur to them to do so or they are uncomfortable asking the proper questions. Physicians, too, are human beings. Patients find talks about sex uncomfortable as well, disclosure of sexual problems embarrassing, and advice sought for sexual fulfillment, hedonistic. But sexual problems are extremely common; *almost everyone experiences a sexual problem or two sometime during his or her life.* When confronting sexual problems and analyzing them, probably the best advice of all (for both patient *and* physician) is to keep in mind Shakespeare's:

"Nothing is right or wrong, but thinking make it so."

Let me tell you a story to illustrate . . . . Several years ago, I encountered a case of sexual dysfunction. A pharmacist came to me for a sperm count. He and his wife were unable to have children and he felt that the proper initial analysis of their problem might be a check on *his* fertility. (Well advised!) His sperm count was normal. A brief history disclosed that this young, healthy, seemingly well-educated male had normal sexual desire, no difficulty in achieving erections, and enjoyed frequent, normal orgasms. Physical examination proved that there was nothing wrong with him: no congenital malformations nor anatomical problems that might suggest a cause for his and his wife's problem.

Next it was his wife's turn for investigation. She too seemed quite normal with respect to libido and ability to reach sexual excitement and orgasm. Her physical examination as well was quite normal.

What to do?

It is said that in cases of infertility, one-third of the time it is the male's problem; one-third of the time, the woman's; and one-third of the time, the couple's together. Was this a case of some rare incompatibility between sperm and vaginal secretions? How might I test for that? Should I launch this couple on an exhaustive infertility workup, to include expensive, intricate anatomical testing of the female anatomy looking for patency of fallopian tubes, normalcy of the uterine cavity, and so forth?

I called them both into the office. They were a handsome couple and, I can remember, held hands during the visit. Nothing wrong there. Offhandedly, and a bit embarrassed, to be sure, I asked them as casually as I could manage how they performed sexual intercourse. He was quite comfortable in his reply.

"Like anyone else, I suppose. I place my penis between her legs and against her clitoris and we hold each other and both move until we have an orgasm."

I tried to hide my disbelief! This couple had, in short, an unconsummated marriage. He had never achieved vaginal penetration and not, it seemed, because of an imperforate, rigid hymen, or pain, or bizarre psychological aversion. The reason seemed to be a simple lack of information. How could a man have graduated from pharmacy school so ill-informed about sexual matters? They were an extremely religious couple, neither of whom had had any sexual experiences before marriage. Neither felt it necessary to acquire any objective sexual education. They simply did what for them came naturally, and for them what came naturally did not include vaginal intercourse. *With the proper information in hand, pregnancy soon followed.*

This type of sexual problem is extremely rare and, for me, was almost unbelievable. The lessons are clear: Sex education is extremely important. Moreover, frank, open discussion of sexual problems is never harmful, and is often beneficial.

Male Sexual Dysfunction

In making the distinction between physical and psychological causes of sexual problems in a man, it is useful to remember some very important differences. *Psychological* causes of sexual dysfunction in the male usually occur *abruptly* and are related to some specific cause which can be found, such as stress, marital difficulties, or the initiation of a certain drug or medicine. *Physical* causes on the other hand are usually *insidious* in onset; the man cannot precisely define when the problem occurred. Psychological causes of sexual dysfunction tend to be intermittent, transient, and episodic. Psychological causes come and go, in other words, whereas physical causes persist and get progressively worse. Men who have psychological problems with impotence or loss of libido generally have the normal erection during the night when sleeping or on first awakening in the morning. Those with physical causes for their dysfunction usually have absence of this normal nocturnal or morning erection.

In the usual medical practice, a male patient most commonly has preserved sexual desire but loss of potency. He rather reluctantly volunteers a decreased ability to achieve erection, but readily admits to normal desire. And, most commonly, the problem can be related to drugs or medications. To say it another way, most sexual dysfunction in a male is because of impotence and most of that can be related to physical causes, specifically drug therapy.

The most common drugs causing impotence in the male are drugs used to treat high blood pressure. Pharmaceutical companies repeatedly make the claim that *their* drug *never* causes sexual problems in the patient. Don't believe it! I have yet to find a drug for high blood pressure that does not in some patient or other cause some degree of impotence. Whether your medication is a beta blocker such as propranolol or a diuretic such as hydrochlorothiazide, if you are man with high blood pressure and on medication and you experience problems of impotence, it is certainly worth mentioning to your physician. He will first want to alter your medications in an effort to restore your sexual performance and get rid of your problem.

Other Drugs Causing Impotence

Alcohol is a frequent culprit in problems of sexual dysfunction. Shakespeare, (Macbeth this time): "It provokes the desire but takes away the performance."

Consumption of alcohol, even without alcoholic intoxication, suppresses a man's ability to achieve erection (and there is no greater way to dampen the desire of a woman than to breathe upon her an alcoholic breath). Taken to this degree, alcohol produces a reversible effect on male potency. In other words, with elimination of the drug, the problem goes away. But chronic alcoholics face another problem. Chronic consumption of alcohol can affect *both* libido and potency. This happens when direct toxic effects of the alcohol damage the testes and the liver. The resulting high levels in the male bloodstream of naturally occurring female hormones can no longer be removed and "detoxified" by the alcoholic's damaged liver.

I had a patient come to me quite irate, convinced that his previous physician had caused his impotence through the prescription of certain high blood pressure medication. In his early sixties, this man had a normal *desire* for sex, but could not achieve an erection. Nor did he experience any erection at night while asleep or on first awakening in the morning. He had stopped taking his blood pressure medicine because of the assumption on his part that the medication was the cause of his problem. Still, his problem did not go away. He was so convinced, in fact, that the blood pressure medication had robbed him of his sex life that he was even talking about lawsuits. Physical examination disclosed marked atrophy of the testes in this man, commonly found in chronic alcoholics. Alcohol, and not blood pressure medication, had irreversibly shriveled his testes. Finally, at this point, the patient admitted to a long history of alcoholism, although he had been sober for several years.

The effect tranquilizers have on sexuality is a complex one. Where anxiety *causes* sexual dysfunction, minor doses of tranquilizers such as Librium or Valium may enhance sexual performance. On the other hand, if sexual function has been normal before the initiation of such drugs, and abnormal after taking them, the drugs themselves may well be the culprit. Other psychoactive drugs such as antidepressants (imipramine, amitriptyline, Elavil, and others) may also produce sexual dysfunction.

Drugs used to treat gastrointestinal disorders sometimes produce sexual dysfunction in both sexes. Certain medicines used to treat bowel spasms in patients with colitis or ulcer disease can cause both impotence and loss of libido in both sexes. With these drugs women may experience a decrease in vaginal lubrication as well as a problem with sexual arousal. Men may experience difficulty in achieving erection. Cimetidine or Tagamet, a new drug used to treat ulcer disease, is a recognized cause of impotence.

Antihistamines can depress libido and, through decreased vaginal lubrication and inability to achieve erection, interfere with sexual excitement. Digitalis (digoxin, Lanoxin, others) used in heart disease can cause impotence in the male as well as occasionally causing male breast enlargement.

Whether cigarette smoking causes sexual dysfunction is debatable. (It probably does not, even though I would like to say it does, because I would like you to stop smoking. And tobacco-breath also dampens the ardor of many people.) But there is no question that chronic marijuana use is associated with impotency and, in some male smokers, breast enlargement as well. Some very good scientific studies show a decrease in male hormone (testosterone) in frequent marijuana users.

Other Physical Causes of Impotence in the Male

Patients with coronary artery disease and angina pectoris may avoid sex because it precipitates chest pain. Newer drug treatment for angina (see Chapter Nine) can avoid this problem. Diabetes mellitus, with its circulatory problems (discussed in Chapter Five), not infrequently has attendant sexual dysfunction, especially in the male. Most estimates of the frequency of sexual dysfunction in male diabetics place it at about fifty percent; one out of every two men with diabetes has problems with sexual performance. Usually the problems of sexual dysfunction occur years after the diagnosis of diabetes, but occasionally a problem of impotence may actually lead the doctor to the diagnosis of diabetes mellitus. The impotence in diabetes has its cause principally in diabetes' effect on the nerves of the body. There is good medical evidence that diabetics who poorly control their disease are more likely to develop this type of nerve damage. The best treatment then is prevention — this means close attention to diet and drug control of blood sugars in the diabetic.

In elderly men, prostate problems may lead to problems of potency. Enlargement of the prostate per se does not. But when the prostate enlarges so greatly as to necessitate surgical removal of part of it, the surgery may result in sexual dysfunction. Most commonly, surgical removal of the prostate by way of an instrument inserted through the penile urethra does not result in any change in sexual function. Total removal of the prostate through an abdominal operation almost always *does*. Inflammation or infection of the prostate, called prostatitis, can give rise to pain on erection and ejaculation, and so indirectly temporarily affect desire or libido. Such prostatic infections are easily treated with antibiotics.

Psychological Causes of Male Sexual Dysfunction

In a young man, sexual dysfunction is almost always because of psychological reasons. The reasons are profound, and beyond the scope of this book. It is sufficient to say that most of the reasons are treatable and in most instances normal sexual function can be restored.

Premature ejaculation is a common problem in young men. There are a whole host of pscychological reasons for it: fear of performance, infrequent orgasm, hostility toward or distrust of the sexual partner, poor self-esteem, or profound marital problems. Treatment of premature ejaculation must address the cause, especially in the case of marital conflict. In some instances, continued sexual experience is all that is necessary. In other cases, the simple treatment outlined in *Human Sexual Inadequacy* (see bibliography) is extremely effective. The same psychological causes for premature ejaculation may cause decreased libido or difficulty in achieving an erection. It is not difficult to understand how guilt, anxiety, depression, and marital strife, not to mention job stress and the vicissitudes of life, can interfere with male performance.

Sexual Dysfunction in the Woman

When we speak of impotence we usually think of the man. But in considering inhibited sexual excitement, it is easy to understand a woman's normal sexual desire dampened, for example, because of pain on intercourse. Indeed the most frequent cause of inhibited sexual excitement in the woman is vaginal irritation from some cause or other: one of the infections we have examined above, for example — candidiasis, trichomoniasis, or bacterial infection — or in the postmenopausal woman, thinning and drying of the vaginal tissues, so-called **atrophic vaginitis.** Atrophic vaginitis in the postmenopausal woman does cause inhibition of sexual excitement but women seldom mention it, surprisingly. It is almost always successfully treated with the application of estrogen creams. A curious complication may result, however.

A long-time patient of mine complained of pain on intercourse. She was postmenopausal. Her physical examination demonstrated drying and thinning of the vaginal tissues, i.e. atrophic vaginitis, and I prescribed for her a certain estrogen cream. Her problem became worse. Using an office nurse as an intermediary, I instructed her to continue trying the cream. Again, through the nurse as an intermediary, I learned that her problem was no better, and instead was getting progressively more severe. She called and left a message that she had to stop using the cream because it was making her problem so much more severe. I instructed her to come into the office.

Examination disclosed marked swelling and redness of the vaginal tissues. She had an obvious allergic reaction to the carrier-cream containing the estrogen medication. Another type of cream was tried, and then another, before we found a cream to which she was not allergic.

Another common sexual dysfunction in the woman is **vaginismus.** This, an involuntary contraction of the vaginal muscles at the outer part of the vaginal outlet, has a physical result but often a psychological cause. The muscles may contract involuntarily because of pain experienced with vaginal penetration, pain because of vaginal infection or irritation, or because of an intact hymen for example. However, more commonly vaginismus occurs as a result of a psychogenic cause. Negative feelings about sex, sometimes engendered through religious orthodoxy, or, more uncommonly, severe traumatic sexual experiences, may give rise to vaginismus. Treatment of the problem must get at the cause and, except in severe traumatic experiences on the part of the woman, treatment of vaginismus is almost always successful.

Orgasmic dysfunction in women is becoming less common today due in large measure to the liberation of women, sexual and otherwise. Men have always had society's permission to be sexual creatures; women only recently so.

Several of the drugs discussed in the section on male sexual dysfunction can affect a woman's sexual desire as well. Nor are women immune to the effects of alcohol. A woman who is a closet alcoholic may have sexual dysfunction as her first symptom of alcoholism. Her partner's objectivity, and compassion, are extremely important for effective treatment.

The DINS Syndrome

A patient of mine had a hysterectomy for malignant disease. She came to me because of a decrease in her sex drive, as perceived both by her and by her husband. She wondered whether the hysterectomy itself had caused a "hormonal problem," affecting her sex drive. Some women, in fact, feel "less female" after hysterectomy and this feeling can affect libido. I discussed this with her. It did not seem to be her problem. Nor was she on any medication which might affect her sex drive. Close questioning revealed that she had experienced a decrease in her libido well *before* her hysterectomy.

About a year before, she had opened a shop of her own, often putting in twelve hour days to ensure its success. After these long working days, she would return home to the typical second-job often relegated to women, that of caring for her family. She was simply worn out, over-worked, fatigued. This was the basis for her decreased libido. So common is this syndrome in the day of the working woman that it has been given a name: the DINS syndrome! (Double Income No Sex).

Psycho-Sexual Dysfunction — A Summary

Masters and Johnson have best summarized the psychological issues surrounding sexual dysfunction:

- It is not useful to blame one's partner or oneself for the occurrence of a sexual problem.
- There is no such thing as an uninvolved partner when sexual difficulties exist.
- Sexual dysfunctions are common problems and do not usually indicate psychopathology.
- It is not always possible to be certain of the precise origin of a sexual dysfunction, but treatment can frequently proceed successfully even when such knowledge is lacking.
- In general, cultural stereotypes about how men and women should behave or function sexually are misleading and counterproductive.
- Sex is not something a man does to a woman or for a woman. It is something a man and woman do together.
- Sex does not only mean intercourse; apart from procreative purposes there is nothing inherent in coitus that makes it always more exciting, more gratifying, or more valuable than other forms of physical contact.
- Sex can be a form of interpersonal communication at a highly intimate level; when sexual communications are not satisfactory, it often indicates that other aspects of a relationship might benefit from enhanced communication as well.
- Using past feelings or behaviors to predict the present is not likely to be helpful since such predictions tend to become self-fulfilling prophecies or limit the freedom to change.
- Developing awareness of one's feelings and the ability to communicate feelings and needs to one's partner sets the stage for effective sexual interaction.

• Assuming responsibility for oneself rather than delegating this responsibility to one's partner is often an effective means of improving the sexual relationship.

CONTRA-CEPTION

Let's talk about condoms. Condoms are a great way to prevent pregnancy and practice safe sex at the same time. But consider a few provisos! Condoms made from lamb intestine (Naturalamb, others) are *not* impervious to viruses. Condoms made of latex rubber are a better idea if you are interested in avoiding AIDS, which is an even better idea! Condoms coated with nonoxynol-9 offer protection against pregnancy if the condom leaks. In addition to protecting against infection with AIDS, condoms obviously protect against other sexually transmitted diseases as well.

There is a problem with condoms. The size of the penis decreases after orgasm. Therefore, after orgasm, a condom fits less well. If vaginal penetration persists for very long after orgasm, the ill-fitting condom may leak around the top. Pregnancy can result.

Intrauterine devices (IUD's) are an effective means of contraception. How they work may be an important consideration to some women for religious reasons. They cause a "mini-abortion." The egg, or ovum, released from the ovary is, it should be remembered, fertilized in the fallopian tube. When the fertilized egg reaches the uterine cavity containing an intrauterine device, the developing egg, not yet an embryo, cannot implant upon the uterus and so is aborted. Intrauterine devices have an increased risk of uterine infection and infection of the fallopian tubes as well. Because of this risk of pelvic infection, infertility can be a side effect of intrauterine devices. IUD's are generally not recommended if a woman plans to have more children.

Diaphragms and cervical caps, used together with vaginal spermicides, theoretically have a high degree of success in preventing pregnancy. Practically, the failure rate is higher than that for condoms and much higher than that for IUD's or birth control pills.

Oral Contraceptives

The pill remains highly effective. Its failure rate is lower than for any other form of contraception. However, birth control pills have their problems. There is an increased risk of formation of blood clots: thrombosis and embolism. For this reason those oral contraceptives which contain *no more than 35 micrograms* of estrogen are preferred. Remember also that some breast cancers are estrogen-dependent; that is, their continued growth depends upon the availability of estrogen. The more estrogen, the faster the growth. This does *not* mean that birth control pills *cause* breast cancer. There is *no* evidence for that. It does mean that monthly breast self-examination and yearly breast examination by your physician, with mammograms as appropriate, as outlined in Chapter Ten, should always be the rule.

If you have a history of blood clots in the veins, don't take the pill. If you have a history of severe migraine attacks, you may have a risk for stroke if you take the pill. Discuss this point with your doctor. If you have difficulty controlling your blood pressure, birth control pills may make that problem worse. Discuss *this* with your physician. Always start with the lowest amount of estrogen you can get away with. You may have a problem with breakthrough bleeding (bleeding in between your normal periods) — this will necessitate an increase in the dosage of estrogen. But start low. Remember surveillance for breast cancer. In fact, whether you take the pill or not, *remember that point.* And remember too, birth control pills alone will not prevent AIDS.

Periodic abstinence as a form of birth control is widely practiced. One avoids coitus during times of highest risk for pregnancy. The failure rate for this technique is the highest of any method of contraception, even under optimal conditions (that is, absolutely regular menstrual cycles).

In many countries, intramuscular injections of a progesterone compound every three months or so are used as a very effective form of contraception. These shots are as effective in preventing pregnancy as is a tubal ligation. The medicine (Depo-Provera) is available in the United States but, as of this writing, it is not approved by the FDA for contraception. There is some evidence that it may cause breast cancers. The soundest advice at present is *not* to use this method of birth control.

Vasectomy for the male is an office surgical procedure. Under local anesthesia, the scrotum is entered and the tubes normally conducting sperm from the testes to the urethra are divided and tied off. Vasectomy is relatively free of complications. The early scare that vasectomy was associated with an increased risk of developing coronary disease is unfounded. Tubal ligation for the woman means day surgery — the complication rate here is also extremely low. General anesthesia is used. The fallopian tubes are then cut and tied off, preventing the ovum from uniting with sperm. Although both are "permanent" forms of contraception, tubal ligation can often be successfully reversed. Vasectomy is far less successfully reversed.

Discuss contraception with your teenagers. That bears repeating. I have had patients, teenagers, who have attempted to practice birth control in many ways:

- Inserted an oral contraceptive pill vaginally in an effort to practice birth control. (It won't work!)
- Douched with Coca Cola after intercourse as a birth control measure. (Doesn't work either!)
- Worried needlessly about pregnancy after having had oral sex.
- Worn a diaphragm for *days* after a single sexual encounter, for fear of pregnancy. (The result was an infection.)

CONCLUSION

The most important message of this chapter is this: Sex education should be *the top priority* in health education. For both patient and physician, that should be a primary concern. Also, when considering sexually transmitted diseases, remember the message in Chapter Twelve: No disease, not AIDS nor any other, carries with it any moral judgment. Be willing to discuss problems of sexual dysfunction with your physician. That is the best place to start. Starting with a "sex counselor" is like going to a cardiovascular surgeon to get an evaluation for chest pain. Explore these problems with your own private physician. And, finally, never take a written prescription on face value. *Ask questions about prescribed drugs,* birth control pills or otherwise, and fully understand, as best you can, how they work and what their side effects might be.

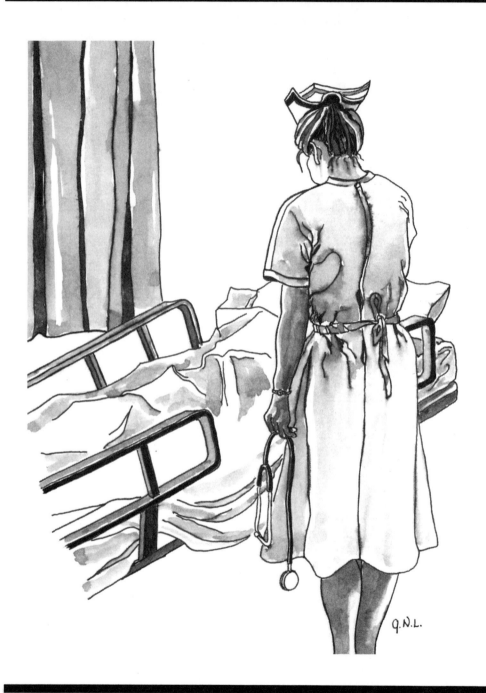

14

How to Live and How to Die

"For everything there is a season, and a time for every purpose under heaven: a time to be born, and a time to die; a time to plant, and a time to pluck up that which is planted; a time to kill, and a time to heal; a time to break down, and a time to build up; a time to weep and a time to laugh; a time to mourn, and a time to dance. A time to cast away stones, and a time to gather stones together; a time to embrace and a time to refrain from embracing; a time to seek, and a time to lose; a time to keep, and a time to cast away. A time to rend and a time to sew; a time to keep silence, and a time to speak; a time to love and a time to hate; a time for war, and a time for peace."

Ecclesiastes 3:1-8

A VIEW OF LIFE

Two men worked in a mill. Everyday at noon they would take their lunch boxes and sit out in the millyard, watching the pulpwood being craned from the trucks and the smoke billowing from the smokestacks. They rarely talked to each other. Each would open his lunch bucket, take out sandwich and coffee, and munch away, quietly surveying the scene.

This went on for twenty years.

One day while unpacking his lunch, the first man said to the second, "Oh no! Peanut butter again!"

"Who makes your lunch?" asked the second man.

"I do," said the first man.

Who makes *your* lunch? Whom will you blame for the tedium of the past twenty years? And even if you *are* one of those uncommon individuals who takes full responsibility for your life, how well are you doing? What is the form of your life? If you have decided upon a form centered around money and the acquisition of property, then the content of your life will necessarily be filled with investing, increasing, and worrying about that money. And if, in the end, you are disenchanted with your life, you will have only yourself to blame. We are all responsible for the form and content of our lives, *for the packing of our own lunches.*

Many have written eloquently about the form a life should take. Their works are listed in the bibliography. One such suggestion of form is worthy of close inspection, because it is both amusing and a lesson on what *not* to do.

In order to better himself, Benjamin Franklin made a list of desirable human attributes. He charted thirteen virtues: temperance, silence, order, resolution, frugality, industry, sincerity, justice, moderation, cleanliness, tranquility, chastity, and humility. His idea was to concentrate on one virtue at a time, striving to become a master of that quality before moving on to the next.

Franklin made charts of the days of the week plotted together with his thirteen virtues. On these charts he rated himself according to how well he lived up to that virtue he was concentrating upon. Each time he transgressed a particular virtue, he would mark a black spot in the appropriate place on his chart.

At the beginning of the next week, he would add a second virtue, silence for example, and would spend that week trying to be both silent and temperate as well. He found that as he concentrated on a second or third virtue, he would become lax with the preceding one, adding more black spots to his performance ratings for previous virtues. He rated himself in this way, working upon his character, for quite some time; and by all that history can tell us, there is every indication that he was reasonably successful.

I am not sure that this is the way for the rest of us. Perhaps we should leave it to the Ben Franklins of the world. Aspirations for sainthood are usually doomed to failure.

But if we are interested in how to live, then we do need to decide upon a form. Karl Menninger and C. S. Lewis have some excellent ideas. I will offer you my idea of one such form.

Christmas Spirit   It is human nature to be oblivious to the misery around us. Without an exercise of denial, how could we possibly retain our sanity in the face of the world's starvation, war, the news from Uganda? We must insulate ourselves from the great horror that life can be. And so, we surround ourselves with illusion, withdrawing from a reality which might otherwise drive us mad. In our illusory world we catch only glimpses of what really goes on around us. Some would say that those who cannot retreat, cannot deny, cannot insulate, who always see our world as it really is, have as their only alternative, psychosis.

When we see the hardships of the "have nots" juxtaposed with the indifference of the "haves," we should not condemn our heartlessness, but rather marvel at our ability for self-deception. It is in the very nature of things. It is existential.

To contend, we exercise a "waiting for Godot." We embroil ourselves in ritual. It is my belief that the greater our power of awareness, the more elaborate our rituals must be. But in *every* life there is ritual and illusion nevertheless. The nature of the ritual (and the form of our lives) is the one great characteristic which sorts us out one from the other. And the one great distinguishing virtue is courage.

For many people, the ritual of life can be quite simple: eight hours at a mill with lunch, then supper, four hours of television, and finally, sleep. Intermingled with this kind of life is a sense of helplessness, and of powerlessness. What could *I* possibly do? What could *I* possibly give? Interwoven too is a sense of guilt, from never trying, or from having failed — the deep guilt of having touched no one else.

As one's business day becomes more frenzied, intellectual awareness more acute, life more sophisticated, ritual grows more elaborate. Those with power and money may discharge their obligations to the welfare of man through taxes, donations, and repetitive prayer. But are these measures, though intrinsically good in themselves, enough? Do they represent any real involvement, or is there, in all honesty, an underlying apathy? When we give a few dollars during the collection at Sunday service, how many lives have we really changed for the better?

Our illusions are maintained in our intellectual life as well. We complain and criticize; we meet and discuss. We form action committees. We study the situation. We spend millions establishing a bureaucracy, believing it will help people. Convinced that our own actions can have no cosmic significance, we feel that we can at least complain about the way things are, and in that complaining, we begin to believe we have solved matters.

Such apathy and denial are normal; it is human nature. We must divorce ourselves from a full comprehension of human suffering in order to live our own lives. *How often we let down our guard to look at reality, how much we see, and what we do about it has to do with courage.* It is also in the nature of things that some people will have more courage than others. Courage is not simply a question of intrinsic virtue. One is endowed with more or less of it. Very occasionally, once in a generation or so, a true hero emerges, taking large bites of reality, assimilating them, and plunging into remarkable solutions. And the world is given an Albert Schweitzer. The rest of us seem to vacillate between velleity and resolve.

Is it any wonder that Christmastime is so often marked by feelings of depression and emptiness? At a time of year when miracles once happened, when all things were once possible, the splashes of red and green all too often turn to gray. We do struggle for the Christmas spirit. And maybe with a surfaced memory, a favorite carol, or the purchase of a thoughtful gift, one feels that spirit: a sudden suffusion of power, of selflessness, of heroism. For a moment we transcend.

And just as suddenly, the feeling is gone. A palpable, vague, unexplained guilt remains. Something is missing. We feel that there should be more. The loss of our traditional society, of our extended families, of the ease of large gatherings, only adds to our isolation and deepens our apathy.

At a time when we should *all* become heroes, we add instead more ritual. We get out the Christmas cards. We shop, put up the lights, and shop some more. We decorate the tree, phone the relatives, and do more shopping. And finally it's done; we've gotten through another Christmas. Lacking a courage to create, subliminally aware of the empty Christmases around us, failing to be the heroes we had always intended to be, we can only wonder what it is that's missing.

Frank Herbert, in *DUNE,* said:

> *No matter how exotic human civilization becomes, no matter the developments of life and society nor the complexity of the machine/human interface, there always come interludes of lonely power when the course of human-kind, the very future of human-kind, depends upon the relatively simple actions of single individuals.*

Could there be a better suggestion for a form to life? One

may harness this Christmas spirit, use it to transcend
intention, and from it fuel our courage. We may use this
spirit to plunge into reality, and take action. Though
such action may be viewed as aberrant behavior at any
other time of year, we can, if we start at Christmas, be
blamed only for 'an excess of Christmas spirit.' We can
seek out those who need us, rather than wait to be
instructed. Fortified by the collective spirit of the time,
we can create out of a collective courage. We may shy
away from carolling alone, but we can certainly carol
together. Forgetting for a time that government, taxes,
welfare, and Medicaid are today's solutions, we could
begin to supply some solutions of our own. We can give.
We may never feed Uganda, but we can try. And with
effort, considerable effort, *we can make this largess of
spirit a habit year-round.*

HOW TO DIE

In twenty years of medicine any physician meets Death
all too frequently. We see patients, in the process of
dying, consumed with anger, or self-pity, preoccupied
with denial to the end, or, occasionally, filled with a
sense of serenity one can only wonder at. From my
experience, certain truths emerge:

- Patients for whom family has been part of the form
  of their lives have a far easier time contending
  with death.
- The more unhappy the marriage, the more violent
  the remaining spouse's reaction to death.
- Those patients with strong religious beliefs have
  an easier time of it. Any doctor, caring for a dying
  patient, will be relieved to know that religion is a
  large part of the form and content of his patient's
  life.
- Dying patients who have never experienced suffering in themselves or in others are more easily
  prone to self-pity.
- Dying patients invariably experience a great
  amount of guilt, especially for this involuntary
  hardship they feel they themselves have caused
  for their families and friends.

What can we make of this? Are there any guidelines we can use in helping someone die? I believe there are.

The Doctor's Role

The doctor is the only person relating to the dying patient who *cannot* be expected to spend long periods of time engaged with the patient in contemplation and consolation. For one thing, the doctor will be far too busy in his or her practice to be expected to perform this function. For another, the physician will usually have other dying patients. To become so committed to all of these dying patients would be both physically and emotionally impossible. What is the doctor's role for the dying patient? That role is not well defined. Most simply stated, *the physician's role is to be available.*

Perhaps the dying patient will be a young girl. Over the months of her illness, she will demand more and more of her parents' time and energy. Her parents will feel an understandable anger and impatience at these incessant demands, and a guilt over this anger, a guilt from neglecting the rest of the family, the other children. It will be the doctor's role to assuage this guilt, to explain its naturalness, to help the family construct a tolerable mode of living within the framework of the dying process. Or, the young girl, the dying patient, will experience pain, or an intolerance to certain foods, or an inability to sleep, or inordinate fear. The physician's role will be to relieve pain and discomfort, to reassure the family, to answer questions, and to interpret the fears.

The Role of Family

The most important person for the dying patient is the spouse, given a pre-existing committed relationship. And the most important role a spouse can perform for the dying patient is to let the dying patient talk about his or her disease. If the patient wallows in self-pity, as most patients will from time to time, he or she should be encouraged to talk about those feelings to the spouse. The spouse in fact should elicit from the patient those feelings of self-pity. Talking about feelings is always helpful to the patient. And when the patient feels guilt over having introduced this hardship into the family, the spouse should encourage expression of that guilt. The spouse should anticipate the depression, denial, anger, self-pity, and acceptance that are the normal stages of the dying process. It is the *spouse,* and *not* the patient, who should get counseling, psychotherapy, moral support, *whatever* is required to help contend with the patient's illness. The patient no longer needs this kind of support; the patient needs the spouse's love and understanding. The spouse needs strength and support to continue to cope with the patient's illness.

If there is no spouse, the next best therapist for the dying patient is a close friend. A friend performs this role far better than does a minister, whose attentions are diffused, whose time is limited, whose attachment is less intimate. Likewise, a doctor cannot adequately perform this role. There is strength as well, and a source of consolation, from groups, especially for those patients who are terminally ill and who are in the process of dying over months or years, such as those patients with AIDS, breast cancers, or certain leukemias. Because of shared experience and shared emotions, groups of terminally ill patients can be extremely helpful for the dying patient.

The Role of Planning

The patient and spouse or friend should discuss the everyday mechanics of life. Money, vacations, and all unfinished business should be openly discussed. Too often spouses and friends exercise so much denial that unfinished business never gets done. This lack of attention to practical matters can have disastrous consequences for those left behind.

The dramatic last trip should be viewed with skepticism. These trips take the form of "I want to see the Alps one last time," or "if I could just see the South Pacific . . . just once . . ." and so on. Usually such trips are disasters. The dying patient is already too compromised in health to enjoy the trip and too preoccupied with dying to profit from the experience. The dramatic last trip ends up simply wasting money.

Never plan ahead more than about six to eight

weeks. You will avoid disappointment. Anything that decreases a patient's burden will make dying easier. If, for example, an AIDS patient is expected to die within the year and a grand family reunion is planned three months hence, the desire to appear healthy and reasonably presentable can become an intolerable psychological burden for the patient. Living day-to-day is best.

The Role of Guilt It can never be stressed too strongly how guilty a patient feels for his or her own illness. The patient, now extremely sensitive to others, sees the sadness in his family and the burden to his friends his illness has caused. Anything that lessens that guilt, whether it is acceptance of the illness on the part of the family and friends, or an open discussion of the patient's guilt and its ill-founded nature, will be of help to the patient. Conversely, anything that increases that guilt adds to the patient's suffering.

I will warn you about one such popular movement which does promote guilt and increases suffering. That is the widely held notion that a patient is *responsible* for his or her own terminal illness. The propaganda goes something like this: If a patient has breast cancer, it is because she became depressed, had let down her guard, failed to marshal her own body defenses, and so "allowed" the cancer to come. Or, another way: A patient dying of cancer is expected to marshal his or her own immune response, "image" the body's defenses fighting the cancer. If such "imaging" is successful, it is the patient's doing. If the patient is not successful, and the cancer has its way, it is the patient's fault. *No person should ever be led to believe that he or she is responsible for illness.* A depressed patient may set in motion certain adverse biochemical events. And those events may lead to certain disease processes. That seems to be more and more substantiated. But in some way the power of prayer is related to healing as well. There is so much that we don't understand. We *can* appreciate that nothing is gained by increasing a dying patient's guilt.

The Role of Religion

I am on tenuous ground here. I do not mean to propose that every dying person should be smothered in religion and prayer. I merely propose this — always ask a dying person this question:

"Do you have a religion?"

If the answer is "no," take it at that and leave it alone. Dying people are tortured by do-gooders who assault them with prayer and botched miracles and end up only fomenting anger and despair in the person.

Sometimes, however, the answer to your question will be "yes." And I am always amazed by those patients who seem not to have any religious beliefs, who have not had a minister visiting them daily in the hospital, who seem to have had no spiritual life through the years of my knowing them — I am always amazed at these people, that they feel, though they once had a religion, and would like to have it again, nevertheless *for them it is now too late.*

I recently had such a patient, a man in his sixties who had a rapidly advancing esophageal cancer for which there is usually no effective treatment. In a matter of a few months he had lost fifty pounds and rapidly approached death. I asked him the question, "Do you have a religion?"

"Well, yes and no. I used to have a religion, but I haven't gone for years, and it's too late now. What's the use? They wouldn't welcome me anyway."

"You might give it a try," I answered. "Why don't you have your family call your minister? Maybe he'll stop by. You never know."

A week later, the man's daughter called to tell me that he had died. *He had been baptized the day before.*

The Role of Humor

One last story . . . . Several years ago a close friend of mine, the restaurateur, developed a widespread cancer that would claim him within a year. Through the entire process he never lost his sense of humor. He would, for example, "prefer" his chemotherapy to any coarse Sicilian wine. His hair loss would give him Picasso-like sex appeal. And so on. He and I continued our traditional monthly trips to the Boston restaurants. On one of these occasions, when he was very near the end and obviously ill, showing all of the ravages of surgery, radiation therapy, and chemotherapy, we were waited on by a particularly arrogant waiter. This was the kind of waiter we have all met before, the man with a perpetual sneer, who favored you with his presence after a thirty minute wait, who was the very essence of haughty contempt, who would not "permit" you to order a particular wine because it might "fight" with the Béarnaise.

My friend placed his order with this man, and then looked at him sardonically and said, "I would appreciate prompt service. I am dying of cancer."

¯Bibliography¯

Chapter Two

American Academy of Family Physicians, 1740 W. 92nd Street, Kansas City, Missouri 64114, 1-816-333-9700.

American College of Physicians, 4200 Pine Street, Philadelphia, Pennsylvania.

American Osteopathic Association, 142 East Ontario, Chicago, Illinois 60611, 1-800-621-1773.

Becker, Ernest: *Denial of Death.* Macmillan, New York, 1973.

Chapter Three

Barker, Burton, and Zieve: *Principles of Ambulatory Medicine.* Chapters 1-9, Williams and Wilkins, 1986.

Groves, James E.: "Taking Care of the Hateful Patient," NEW ENGLAND JOURNAL OF MEDICINE, 298 (16):883, 1978.

Jones, J. Alfred, M.D., Phillips, Gerald W.: *Communicating With Your Doctor: Rx for Good Medical Care.* Southern Illinois University Press, June 1988.

Chapter Four

Abbott, C., Starker, J.: "The Ten Healthiest Cities in America," HEALTH 20:31-35, March 1988.

Breslow, L., Sommers, A. R.: "The Lifetime Health-Monitoring Program: A Practical Approach to Preventative Medicine," NEW ENGLAND JOURNAL OF MEDICINE, 296:601, 1977.

Conyers, J., Jr. (D-Mich.): "Dealing with Occupational and Environmental Dangers," USA TODAY 113:91-2, July 1984.

Council on Scientific Affairs, American Medical Association: "Medical Evaluation of Healthy Persons," JAMA 249:1626, 1983.

Fox, M. R.: "Perspectives in Risk," VITAL SPEECHES OF THE DAY 53:730-2, September 15, 1987.

Frame, P. S.: "A Critical Review of Adult Health Maintenance," JOURNAL OF FAMILY PRACTICE 22:341, 417, 511, 23:29, 1986.

Goodman, S.: "The Signs of Life: A Guide to Assessing Your Health Risks," CURRENT HEALTH 13:3-9. April 1987.

Hales, D.: "Who's Got the Good Life?" HEALTH 15:28-31, April 1983.

Kaplan, J., et al.: "Our Bodies, Our World: How the Environment

Affects Our Health," VOGUE 177:402-407, October 1987. (A special section devoted to environmental risks).

Koshland, D. E., et al.: Risk Assessment Issue. SCIENCE 236: April 17, 1987. (An issue devoted to environmental and carcinogenic risks and risk assessment. A highly scientific and impartial review of the problem of risks and risk assessment.)

Medical Practice Committee, American College of Physicians: "Periodic Health Examination: A Guide for Designing Individualized Preventative Health Care in the Asymptomatic Patient," ANNALS OF INTERNAL MEDICINE 95:729, 1981.

Oboler & LaForce: "The Periodic Physical Examination in Asymptomatic Adults," ANNALS OF INTERNAL MEDICINE, Vol. 110, No. 3, February 1, 1989, p. 214.

Peterson, C.: "How Much Risk is Too Much?" SIERRA 70:62-64, May-June 1985.

Resch, T.: "Health Hazards," BLAIR AND KETCHUM'S COUNTRY JOURNAL 13:14-15, January 1986.

Ruckelshaus, W.: "Risk and Society," CONSUMER'S RESEARCH MAGAZINE 67:37-8, June 1984.

Samet & Nero: "Indoor Radon and Lung Cancer," NEW ENGLAND JOURNAL OF MEDICINE, March 2, 1989, p. 591.

Shell, E.: "The Risks of Risk Studies," THE ATLANTIC MONTHLY 260:114-15, November 1987.

Chapter Five

American Diabetes Association, Inc., 1660 Duke Street, Alexandria, Virginia 22314.

American Dietetic Association, 208 S. LaSalle Street, Suite 1100, Chicago, Illinois 60604-1003.

American Heart Association National Center, 7320 Greenville Avenue, Dallas, Texas 75231.

"Detection, Evaluation, and Treatment of High Blood Cholesterol in Adults," The National Cholesterol Education Program, U.S. Department of Health and Human Services Public Health Service, NIH Publication #88-2925, January 1988.

INTERNAL MEDICINE ALERT. Vol. 10, No. 16, August 29, 1988. pp. 61-62.

THE MEDICAL LETTER ON DRUGS AND THERAPEUTICS, Vol. 30 (Issue 774), September 9, 1988, pp. 81-84.

Chapter Six

Bennett, William, M.D. & Gurin, Joel: *The Dieter's Dilemma: Eating Less and Weighing More.* Basic Books, Inc., New York, 1982. (Sound, erudite advice; based on the "set-point" theory of obesity. "How to Write Your Own Diet Book" in Chapter Eight should be read first by anyone tempted by the pulp diet books on the shelves.)

Brody, Jane: *Jane Brody's Nutrition Book.* W. W. Norton & Company, New York, 1981. (The best diet book ever written.)

Kleinfield, N. R.: "Why Hospitals Love Diets," THE NEW YORK TIMES, Sunday, Nov. 6, 1988, p. 4. (In the business section!)

Watson, Richard: *The Philosopher's Diet.* Atlantic Monthly Press, Boston/New York, 1985.

Chapter Seven

Blackburn, Henry and Jacobs, David R., Jr.: "Physical Activity and the Risk of Coronary Heart Disease," NEW ENGLAND JOURNAL OF MEDICINE. November 3, 1988, Vol. 319, #18, p. 1217.

CONSUMER REPORTS. November, 1986.

Cooper, Kenneth H.: *Aerobics.* Bantam Books, New York, 1968.

Cooper, Kenneth H.: *The New Aerobics.* Bantam Books, New York, 1970.

Cooper, Kenneth H. & Mildred: *Aerobics for Women.* Bantam Books, New York, 1972.

Densmore, Frances: *Uses of Plants by the Chippewa Indians.* United States Government Printing Office, Washington, 1928.

Eaton, S. B., Shostak, M., and Konner, M.: *The Paleolithic Prescription.* Harper & Row, New York, 1988.

Fixx, James F.: *The Complete Book of Running.* Random House, New York, 1977.

Fletcher, Colin: *The Complete Walker.* Alfred A. Knopf, New York, 1968.

Kostrubala, Thaddeus: *The Joy of Running.* J. B. Lippincott, Philadelphia, 1976.

PSI - NordicTrack Company, 141 Jonathan Boulevard, N., Chaska, Minnesota 55318.

RUNNERS' WORLD. "The Great Indoors," December, 1988, p. 26.

Ibid. "Who's the fittest?" p. 34.

Simon, Harvey B., M.D., F.A.C.P: *Scientific American Medicine: Current Topics in Medicine: Exercise, Health, and Sports Medicine.* Scientific American, Inc., 1988.

Watson, Richard: *The Philosopher's Diet.* Atlantic Monthly Press, Boston/New York, 1985.

Chapter Eight

Alcoholics Anonymous (The Big Book): Obtained through AA World Services, Box 459, Grand Central Station, New York, New York 10017.

Benowitz, Neal: *Pharmacologic Aspects of Cigarette Smoking and Nicotine Addiction.* NEW ENGLAND JOURNAL OF MEDICINE, Vol. 319, No. 20, November 17, 1988, pp. 318-328. (Excellent discussion with 167 references.)

Clark, William D.: "Alcoholism: Blocks to Diagnosis and Treatment," AMERICAN JOURNAL OF MEDICINE, Vol. 71, August, 1981, p. 275.

"Clinical Opportunities for Smoking Intervention: A Guide for the Busy Physician," National Heart, Lung, and Blood Institute Smoking Education Program, NIH, Bethesda, Maryland 20892, NIH publication #86-2178, August 1986.

Department of Health, Education, and Welfare: "Smoking and Health: A Report of the Surgeon General," Washington, D.C., 1979.

Fielding, Jonathan E.: "Smoking: Health Effects and Control" (two parts), NEW ENGLAND JOURNAL OF MEDICINE, Vol. 313, August 22 & 29, 1985, pp. 491, 555.

The Good Life: A Guide to Becoming an Ex-Smoker (pamphlet). American Heart Association, National Center, 7320 Greenville Avenue, Dallas, Texas 75231 (Free for the asking).

How to Quit: A Guide to Help You Stop Smoking (pamphlet). American Heart Association, National Center, 7320 Greenville Avenue, Dallas, Texas 75231 (Free for the asking).

Klerman, G. L.: "Treatment of Alcoholism," NEW ENGLAND JOURNAL OF MEDICINE, Vol. 320, February 9, 1989, p. 394.

West, Maxwell, et al.: *Alcoholism: UCLA Conference.* ANNALS OF INTERNAL MEDICINE, Vol. 100, March 1984, p. 405.

Whitfield, C. L.: "Advances in Alcoholism and Chemical Dependence," THE AMERICAN JOURNAL OF MEDICINE, Vol. 85, October 1988, p. 465.

Chapter Nine

American Heart Association, National Center, 7320 Greenvile Avenue, Dallas, Texas 75231.

Blackburn, Henry and Jacobs, David R., Jr.: "Physical Activity and the Risk of Coronary Heart Disease," NEW ENGLAND JOURNAL OF MEDICINE. November 3, 1988, Vol. 319, No. 18, p. 1217.

Cooper, K. H.: *The New Aerobics.* Bantam Books, New York, 1970.

Eshleman, Ruthe: *American Heart Association Cookbook.* David McKay Co., Inc., 1984.

Kavanagh, T.: *Heart Attack? Counterattack! Practical Plan for a Healthy Heart.* VanNostrand Reinhold, Ltd., Toronto, 1976.

Mayer, J.: *Overweight: Causes, Cost, and Control.* Englewood Cliffs, New Jersey, Prentice Hall Inc., 1968.

Moser, Marvin: *How You Can Help Your Doctor Treat Your High Blood Pressure.* American Heart Association, 1986.

Pfaffenberger, R. S., Jr.: "Work Activity and Coronary Heart Mortality," NEW ENGLAND JOURNAL OF MEDICINE, Vol. 292, No. 11, 1975, pp. 545-550.

Schmeck, H. M.: "The Revolution in Heart Treatment," THE NEW YORK TIMES MAGAZINE, PART II, October 9, 1988, p. 14.

Selye, H.: *The Stress of Life.* New York, McGraw Hill, 1956.

"The 1988 Report of the Joint National Committee on Detection, Evaluation, and Treatment of High Blood Pressure," United

States Department of Health and Human Services, NIH publication #88-1088, May 1988.

"Understanding Angina," American Heart Association, 1984.

"What Science Knows About AIDS" (A Single Topic Issue), SCIENTIFIC AMERICAN, October 1988.

Chapter Ten

Byrne, Gregory: "Going Far on a B.S.," SCIENCE, Vol. 241, 1988, p. 1764.

DeVita, Helmund, and Rosenberg: *CANCER: Principles in Practice of Oncology.* J. B. Lippincott Company, Philadelphia, 1985.

Federman, et al.: *Scientific American Medicine* (Subtitle: Oncology), Scientific American Inc., 1988.

Holleb and Randers-Pehrson: *Classics in Oncology,* American Cancer Society, Inc., New York, New York, 1987.

"Is a Mastectomy Necessary?" CONSUMER REPORTS, November 1988, p. 732.

Kartner & Ling: "Multi-Drug Resistance in Cancer" SCIENTIFIC AMERICAN, Vol. 260, No. 3, March, 1989, p. 44.

Konner, Melvin: "Civilization's Cancer," THE NEW YORK TIMES MAGAZINE, 1988.

"Participatory Risk Management Criteria Diagnosis of Breast Carcinoma," Medical Mutual Insurance Company of Maine, 1988.

Silberner, Joann: "How to Beat Breast Cancer," U.S. NEWS AND WORLD REPORT, July 11, 1988, p. 52.

Chapter Eleven

Lastavica, et al.: "Rapid Emergence of a Focal Epidemic of Lyme Disease in Coastal Massachusetts," NEW ENGLAND JOURNAL OF MEDICINE, Vol. 320, Jan. 19, 1989, p. 133.

"The Medical Letter on Drugs and Therapeutics," Vol. 30, Issue 780, December 2, 1988, p. 109.

"Watch Out for the Tick Attack," CONSUMER REPORTS, Vol. 54, No. 6, June 1988, p. 382.

Chapter Twelve

"Can You Rely on Condoms?" CONSUMER REPORTS, Vol. 54, No. 3, March, 1989, pp. 135-141.

National AIDS Hotline: 1-800-342-2437.

"Common Questions About AIDS," CONSUMER REPORTS, Vol. 54, No. 3, March 1989, p. 142.

Williams, et al.: "Immunization Policies and Vaccine Coverage Among Adults," ANNALS OF INTERNAL MEDICINE, Vol. 108, No. 4, April 1988, p. 616.

"What Science Knows About AIDS" (A Single Topic Issue), SCIENTIFIC AMERICAN, October 1988.

Chapter Thirteen

"Can You Rely on Condoms?" CONSUMER REPORTS, March, 1989, pp. 135-141.

"Choice of Contraceptives," THE MEDICAL LETTER ON DRUGS AND THERAPEUTICS, Vol. 30, Issue 779, November 18, 1988.

Green, Richard, M.D.: *Human Sexuality: A Health Practitioner's Text*. Williams and Wilkins, Baltimore, 1979.

Kaplan, H. S.: *The Evaluation of Sexual Disorders: Psychological and Medical Aspects*. Brunner/Mazel, New York, 1983.

Kolodny, Masters, Johnson: *Textbook of Sexual Medicine*. Little, Brown & Co., Boston, 1979.

Masters, W. H., Johnson, V.E.: *Human Sexual Inadequacy*. Little, Brown & Co., Boston 1970.

Mishell, D. R.: "Contraception". NEW ENGLAND JOURNAL OF MEDICINE, Vol, 320, No. 12, March 23, 1989, p. 777.

Chapter Fourteen

Campbell, Joseph: *Myths to Live By*. Bantam Books/Viking Penguin, New York, 1972.

Campbell, Joseph: *The Masks of God: Primitive Mythology*. Penguin Books, New York, 1959.

Campbell, Joseph: *The Masks of God: Oriental Mythology*. Penguin Books, New York, 1959.

Campbell, Joseph: *The Masks of God: Occidental Mythology*. Penguin Books, New York, 1959.

Franklin, Benjamin: *Writings*. The Library of America, New York, 1987.

Gold, P. W., Goodwin, F. K. et al.: "Clinical and Biochemical Manifestations of Depression: Relation to the Neurobiology of Stress," NEW ENGLAND JOURNAL OF MEDICINE, Vol. 319, No. 6, August 11 & August 19, 1988, pp. 348, 413.

Jastrow, Robert: *The Enchanted Loom: Mind in the Universe*. Simon & Schuster, New York, 1981.

Jung, C. G.: *Memories, Dreams, Reflections*. Random House, New York, 1965.

Lewis, C. S.: *A Grief Observed*. Bantam Books, New York, 1976.

Lewis, C. S.: *Mere Christianity*. Macmillan, New York, 1943.

Lewis, C. S.: *The Screwtape Letters*. Macmillan, New York, 1982.

Menninger, Karl: *Love Against Hate*. Harcourt, Brace, Jovanovich, New York, 1942.

Menninger, Karl: *Man Against Himself*. Harcourt, Brace, Jovanovich, New York, 1938.

Menninger, Karl: *Whatever Became of Sin?* Bantam Books, New York, 1978.

Peck, M. S.: *The Road Less Traveled*. Simon & Schuster, New York, 1978.

Watson, Richard: *The Philosopher's Diet*. THE ATLANTIC MONTHLY PRESS, Boston, 1985.

Index